Foods That Cause You To Lose Weight

The Negative Calorie Effect

1st Edition, Revised

by Neal Barnard, M.D.

Recipes by Jennifer Raymond

Interior design by Barbara McNew
Printed in the U.S.A.

Twentieth Printing

ISBN 1-882330-31-5

Table of Contents

Introduction

This book offers a new approach to weight control. If your goal is a slimmer body and more energy than you have had in years, this program is more powerful than any diet you have ever tried. It is not a diet. It is a comprehensive program that brings about better weight control than old-fashioned diets ever could.

In this program, we will not compromise. We will use all the factors that are known to promote permanent healthful weight control. You will boost your metabolic rate through food selection, shift your menu from calorie-dense fatty foods to foods with a much better nutrient make-up, and bring in other ways to burn calories more effectively.

This book was written because most diets have not been very successful. Many are simply too weak to get results. Others use an artificial "formula approach" that no one could live with permanently. They may cause a phenomenal weight loss for a few weeks, followed by a huge weight gain back to and beyond the starting point. These frustrating results are caused by the poor design of the diets.

There is a much better way. For years, researchers have used many different kinds of diets to improve health: diets to help people lose weight, lower their cholesterol levels, or deal with various health problems. From these studies, it is clear that there are certain factors which are critical to success in long-term weight control.

For example:

+ Certain foods add easily to fat stores while others do not.
+ Certain foods will alter your metabolism so that calories are burned more effectively.
+ Weight loss should be gradual, not sudden.
+ And, most importantly, a menu that is very low in fat, high in fiber and carbohydrate, and modest in protein, is extraordinarily powerful for weight control.

We will examine these and many other factors in detail.

Old diets focused mainly on quantity. In the new approach used in this program, the type of food that makes up the menu is considerably more important than the quantity of food. In other words, *you can eat until you are full and still lose weight*. No more skimpy portions. If you find that difficult to believe, consider the research. Many clinical studies have examined diets that are based on very small portions and other diets that change the type of food but not the quantity. It turns out that *the type of food you eat is much more important for permanent weight control than the portion size*. In fact, skimpy portion diets can actually impair your ability to burn off calories. Research also shows that thin people actually eat more food, not less, compared to most overweight people. In this program, we will shift the diet toward foods that boost the metabolism and which do not easily add to body fat.

There are also specific factors that make the process of change easier. A diet that brings about long-term success is much more rewarding than one that yields only modest or short-term results. So this program is designed to be as effective as possible.

We will also have opportunities to try new kinds of foods. This is not only fun; it is the critical step in building a new body. Tasting food is when theories about weight control turn into practice. You will learn about specific new foods to try, including menus, recipes, and shopping lists. In addition, we will look at ways to bring in family and friends. They are our allies in life's changes. We will see how to help them help us.

When you put this program to work for you, you can have the slimmest body nature ever intended for you.

How to Use This Program

This program is divided into four parts:

Basic Con- cepts	First, find a comfortable chair and read Part One. In this concise section, you will learn the basic concepts that are essential to a permanent slimming-down program.
Step-by-Step Program	Part Two gets you started with a step-by-step program, including new foods to try, and recipes, and a simple program for physical activity. You can easily chart your progress.
Keeping It Off	Part Three moves the program into high gear, with more advanced information to solidify your gains.
Menus & Recipes	Part Four gives you many more health-ful recipes to make eating a joy.

Get all you can out of this program. No corners were cut in bringing this information to you; do not cut any corners in putting it into action.

You can succeed. So be patient, and don't rush. It took time for you to gain weight, and it will take time for it to come off again. Overly rapid weight loss can lead to a rebound of weight gain, so let the pounds come off gradually. I think you will be happy with the new you.

Notice

This book is not intended to take the place of medical advice.

✦ If you have any medical condition or are on medication, you should consult your doctor before making any substantial change in your diet. Dietary changes can sometimes change your need for medication or have other important effects.

✦ You should also see your doctor before any substantial increase in your physical activity if you are over forty or have any medical condition.

✦ If you are pregnant or nursing, or if you follow this program strictly for more than three years, then take 3 micrograms supplemental vitamin B_{12} each day.

Part I

Basic Concepts

Basic Concepts

We need to think differently about the approach to losing weight. Forget old-fashioned diets. There are very good reasons why they do not work well. Your body was not designed recently. The human body took shape millions of years ago, long before diets were invented. At that time, the lack of food meant only one thing, starvation; and if the body could not cope with the lack of food, the result was life-threatening. So we have built-in mechanisms to preserve ourselves in the face of low food intake. These defenses are automatically put to work. When you go on a low-calorie diet, you know that you are doing so to lose weight. But your body does not know that. As far as your body is concerned you are starving, and it will trigger a number of biological mechanisms to try and stop you.

To see how to avoid this problem, let's first look at how your body burns calories. The speed at which your body burns calories is called *the metabolic rate*. Some people have a "fast metabolism" and burn lots of calories in a short time. They are likely to stay slim. Other people have a slower metabolic rate and have a harder time staying slim.

Your metabolism is like the rate at which an automobile uses up gas. An idling car uses up some fuel. When the car is moving it uses more, and when it accelerates up a hill it will use a lot more gas.

Our bodies work the same way. We burn some calories even when we are relaxing or asleep because it takes energy to maintain our normal body temperature and to keep our lungs, heart, brain and other organs working. When we engage in activities, the more strenuous they are, the more calories we burn.

Dieting Slows Your Metabolism

The point to remember is that your metabolic rate can be changed. In a period of starvation or dieting, the body slows down the metabolism. The body does not understand the concept of dieting. Remember, as far as your body is concerned, a diet is starvation, and it does not know how long the starvation period will last. So it clings to its fat like a motorist

12

who is running out of gas preserves fuel. Remember the last time you were driving along the highway and suddenly noticed that the gas gauge was below empty? You tried to remember how far below "E" your gauge will go. You went easy on the accelerator, driving very smoothly, and turned off the engine at stop lights to conserve gas until you got to a station.

Your body does the same sort of thing when food is in short supply. It turns down the metabolic flame to save as much of the fat on your body as possible until the starvation period is over, because fat is the body's fuel reserve. This is very frustrating to dieters. They often find that, even though they are eating very little, their bodies do not easily shed the pounds. Even worse, the slowed metabolism can continue beyond the dieting period, sometimes for weeks, according to studies at the University of Pennsylvania and elsewhere.[1] For that reason, fat is easily and rapidly accumulated again after the dieting period. This causes the familiar yo-yo phenomenon, in which dieters lose some weight, then rebound to a higher weight than they started with.

Here is the first step to keeping your metabolic rate up: Make sure that your diet contains at least 10 calories per pound of your ideal body weight. This means that if you are aiming for a weight of 150 pounds, your daily menu should contain at least 1500 calories. Weight loss will be gradual, but you will not slow your metabolism and, so, you will be able to retain your progress.

Minimum Calories per day

Ideal Weight x 10 calories = Calories

120 x 10 calories = 1200 Calories
150 x 10 calories = 1500 Calories
180 x 10 calories = 1800 Calories

Avoiding Binges

There is another problem with skimpy eating. Not only does the body lower its metabolic flame to conserve energy; it also gets ready to take maximal advantage of any food source it finds. When food becomes available, there is a tremendous tendency to binge, in what is known as the *"restrained-eater"* phenomenon. You know the pattern. You have been dieting for several days, and suddenly someone brings home a carton of ice cream. A little bit won't hurt, you decide, and before you know it you are scraping the bottom of the carton and digging around the cracks for every last bit. You then scold yourself for your "lack of will power."

The point to remember is binges come from diets.

The truth is that the problem was not will power at all, but, rather, the innate biological programming of the human body. The diet turned on the "anti-starvation" plan that is built into every human being. Your body assumed that any food in front of you might be the only calorie source you might have for a while, so it demanded a binge.

It is not a question of weak will or gluttony. The human body has a built-in tendency to binge after periods of starvation.

For a similar reason, it is best not to skip meals. Skipping breakfast and lunch leads to overeating later in the day. So, eat regular meals and avoid very-low-calorie diets.

Bulimia—binge-eating often followed by purging—almost always begins with a diet. And as the binging begins, shame and secrecy often follow. If this has happened to you, remember that binging is not a moral failing. It is a natural biological consequence of dieting.

Dieting is now a nearly universal pastime in America, and bulimia is an ever-growing epidemic. Unfortunately, children are raised on a menu that is almost certain to make many of them gain weight. The cultural trend in Western countries in the past several decades has emphasized meat, dairy products, fried; chicken, french fries and other high-fat foods. Combined with an increasingly sedentary lifestyle, the predictable result is that many people will become overweight. They mistakenly believe that the problem is the *quantity* of food they are eating, rather than the *type* of food. Rather than abandon the offending foods, they simply eat less. A restrictive diet begins. The natural result is lowered metabolic rates, cravings and binging. Most binges would probably never occur if dieting were replaced with better food choices which would promote a slow, steady drop in weight, rather than an overly rapid weight loss.

Skipped meals and skimpy portions are not effective for permanent weight control and are not a part of this program.

An Optimal Weight-loss Menu

Now that you know what not to do, let's build a program that takes pounds off and keeps them off. The basis of this program is a way of eating that promotes weight control naturally, without counting calories and without skimpy portions.

Let's first look at *carbohydrates*. The starchy white inside of a potato is mostly complex carbohydrate, which is simply a chemist's term for molecules made up of many natural sugars linked together. When you eat a potato, that carbohydrate is gradually broken apart into simple sugars, which are absorbed and used by the body. Rice, wheat, oats, and other grains are rich in complex carbohydrates, as are beans and nearly all vegetables.

In the past, many people believed that starchy foods were fattening. They would avoid carbohydrate-rich potatoes, rice, bread, and pasta. People would take a baked potato, which has only 95 calories, and top it with a pat or two of butter, and sometimes add sour cream, grated cheese, or bacon bits. As they gained weight, they blamed the potato. But we now know that what was fattening was not the potato, but the greasy toppings that were added to it.

✦ Carbohydrate-rich foods are actually low in calories.
✦ A gram of carbohydrate (about $1/30$ ounce) = 4 calories.

That is why a slice of bread has only 70 calories and an ear of corn only 120. A chicken breast, which contains no carbohydrate, has fully 386 calories. In contrast, starchy foods are low-calorie foods.

Compare that to fatty foods. A gram of fat has nine calories, more than twice the calorie content of carbohydrate. It is only when carbohydrate-rich foods are covered with fatty

16

toppings that lots of calories are added.

Look at how this works with actual foods: You are planning a candlelight dinner for two. A nice spaghetti dinner with some fresh vegetables, perhaps a glass of wine. A one-cup serving of spaghetti topped with $1/2$ cup of tomato sauce has about 200 calories. But if we decided to add ground beef to the sauce, look what happens: the spaghetti dinner suddenly has 365 calories. The fat in ground beef holds a lot of calories.

Let's take another example: A half-cup serving of mashed potatoes has 70 calories. A tablespoon of butter on top adds fully 108 calories. In the process a low-calorie food becomes a high-calorie food. In other words, fatty toppings are high in calories, but the carbohydrate-rich potatoes, spaghetti, bread, etc., are not.

Food and Fatty Toppings

Potato (1 med.) = 95 calories

Potato (1 med.) + Butter (1 Tbs) = 203 calories

Potato (1 med.) + Butter (1 Tbs) + Cheese (1 oz) = 317 calories

---

There may be an advantage to whole unprocessed grains, such as rice, cereal, or corn, as opposed to grain which has been ground up into flour (e.g. bread or pasta). Some evidence shows that we tend to extract more calories from the ground-up varieties, perhaps because the process of "digestion" has been begun for us.

There are other important virtues of carbohydrates. They cannot add *directly* to your fat stores. We do not have any "carbohydrate storage areas" on our bellies or thighs. If the body is to store the energy of carbohydrates in fat, it has to chemically convert the carbohydrate molecules into fat. This process consumes a fair number of calories. As a result:

✦

Calories from carbohydrates
are not as likely to increase body fat
as are the same number of calories from fats.

✦

In addition, *carbohydrates boost your metabolism.* Plant-based meals tend to increase the metabolic rate slightly. Here is how it works: Carbohydrate breaks down in the body to various sugars. Sugars cause insulin to be released which, in turn, leads to the production of two natural hormones, norepinephrine and thryoid hormone (T 3). T 3 and norepinephrine both increase the metabolic rate. The result is more effective calorie burning.[2-5]

Carbohydrates Increase Metabolism

Carbohydrates → Sugar → Insulin

Norepinephrine & T3

Increased Metabolism
(More effective calorie burning)

So starchy foods are naturally low in calories, they cannot be automatically added to body fat, and they help boost your metabolic rate so that calories are burned off a bit faster.

✦ Carbohydrate-rich vegetables, beans, and grains are the best friends of anyone trying to shed some pounds.

Now here is a critical point:

✦ Complex carbohydrates are found only in plants.

Grains, such as bread, spaghetti, and rice are loaded with carbohydrates. Beans and vegetables are also high in carbohydrates. But there are virtually no complex carbohydrates in chicken, fish, beef, pork, eggs, or dairy products. The more animal products you eat, the more you are pushing carbohydrate-rich vegetable foods off your plate. That is one reason why the most effective weight-control programs use vegetarian menus.

There is an added bonus to foods from plants: fiber. Grains, beans, and vegetables contain fiber, which adds texture and makes them filling and satisfying. Fiber is what people used to call roughage, the part of plants that resists digestion in the small intestine. The value of fiber was not appreciated until relatively recently, and so it was often removed by refining methods. The result was white bread instead of whole-grain breads, white rice instead of brown rice, and baked goods that were more densely packed with calories and less satisfying than they would have been had the fiber been left in. Fiber adds a hearty texture to foods but has virtually no calories.

Like complex carbohydrates, fiber is found only in plants. Grains, such as wheat, oats, rye, corn, rice, and the breads, cereals, and other foods that are made from them are loaded with fiber. Vegetables of all kinds and legumes, such as beans, peas, and lentils, are also rich in fiber.

Animal products contain no fiber at all. To the extent that animal products are added to the diet, the fiber content is reduced. Americans now consume only 10-20 grams of fiber per day, on average, which is about half of what we should have. The reason, of course, is the penchant for animal products and refined plant foods, which unfortunately displace the fiber-rich foods. *But do not feel that you must calculate your fiber intake.* When you center your diet on high-carbohydrate foods, such as whole grains, beans, and vegetables, the fiber content of your diet will increase naturally. As you will see in Part II, the result will be meals that are satisfying and filling. When we discuss the value of carbohydrate-rich foods and fiber, you can simplify this by thinking in terms of foods from plants versus animal products. A plant-based diet is rich in carbohydrate and fiber. Animal products are devoid of them. The result is that plant-based diets promote slimness, while Animal products promote overweight.

Charlene:
Beating a Weight Problem

Charlene wanted to lose 30 pounds. In fact, she had wanted to lose these same 30 pounds for several years. She had tried several different diets, including some with formula drinks, and had also tried diet pills. None of these were effective over the long run, although all had seemed to help temporarily. When I met her, she was avoiding all carbohydrates. She skipped breakfast, had yogurt and turkey slices for lunch, and usually ate frozen dietetic meals for dinner. Her weight had been essentially the same for months.

I suggested that, instead of avoiding starchy foods, she make them the center of her diet. Breakfast was to be hot cereal and fruit. At work, she could make lunch from dried soups. For dinner, she was to make a pot of rice, as much as she could eat, or, if she preferred, she could have potatoes or other starchy foods instead. She was also to include vegetables and beans or lentils at dinner. Because this "diet" included a rather large quantity of food, she worried that she might actually gain weight on it. But some rather simple calculations showed that the calorie content of this menu was actually very modest. She lost weight very gradually, but about 10 months later, the 30 extra pounds were gone.

The Negative Calorie Effect

Many people still believe that the number of calories in any given food tells you just how fattening that food is likely to be. For example, a cup of rice has about 220 calories. Three slices of bologna also have 220 calories. So some people assume that these two foods have exactly the same effect on the waistline.

They don't. The very same number of calories coming from bologna and from rice have very different effects. The bologna tends to be fattening, as a general rule, while the rice does not.

Rice does provide calories to run the body's functions. And theoretically it is possible for unused calories from rice to be stored as fat. But it turns out that rice is much less fattening than the same number of calories from bologna, other meats, or other fatty foods. Rice—like other carbohydrate-rich foods—has a way of naturally *reducing* the calories that are available for fat storage.

You might think of this as a "negative calorie effect." One of the most exciting concepts in the science of weight control in many years is the fact that certain foods can actually assist in the *loss* of fat.

By now, it will come as no surprise to you that carbohydrate-rich foods are power foods for weight control. But let's see what the "negative calorie effect" really means. Then, we'll look at 20 foods that encourage this effect and which you can eat freely. In reality there are far more than 20, and by the time you are done with this book, I hope you will have gone far beyond the old-fashioned notion of counting calories and limiting portion size. The key is not how much you eat, but, instead, the types of foods you eat.

When you think of carbohydrate, think, for example, of rice. A rice grain is a seed, designed by nature to start a new rice plant. The starchy white interior of a rice grain consists mainly of complex carbohydrates that nourish the seed as it sprouts and grows. The same is true of beans, potatoes, apples, and many other plants. The starchy carbohydrate interior provides nourishment for the tiny growing plant.

For millions of years, humans and other primates have plucked fruits from trees and roots from the ground and have taken advantage of carbohydrate's capacity to nourish us. What is remarkable is that these foods provide energy with relatively little tendency to cause overweight. In many Asian countries, for example, where rice is still the center of the diet and huge amounts of rice are consumed, people tend to remain slim.

While carbohydrates provide calories for the body, they also have ways of counteracting the storage of some of these calories as fat, and also encourage the burning of stored calories:

First, as we saw earlier, a substantial number of the calories in carbohydrates are used up as carbohydrates are turned to fat. Let me give you some numbers: For every 100 calories of carbohydrate that your body tries to store as fat, 23 are lost in the process of breaking down carbohydrate molecules and building fat molecules from them. That means that, of the 220 calories in a cup of rice, about 50 calories are used up just in the chemical processing. Leaving grains whole, like rice, cereals, or corn, rather than grinding them into flour to make bread or pasta, also causes them to release fewer calories.

But that is just the beginning. In addition, because carbohydrate increases the body's metabolism, more calories are burned off as the metabolism increases. The metabolism-boosting effect causes more of the calories in *all the foods you eat* to be burned. When that happens, they cannot be turned into fat.

It is similar to the effect of turning up a car's idle. More gas is used up; there is less in the tank, less to spill on the ground, and less to use in the future, because it has been burned.

Another part of the "negative calorie effect" of carbohydrates is that they are the part of the diet that tells the body when it has had enough food. Your body does not just pay attention to how much you have eaten. It actually has a way to monitor how much carbohydrate is coming in. When it has had enough, it reduces the feeling of hunger. Carbohydrates are the cue the body needs. So, if there is a lot of carbohydrate on your plate, you will tend to eat to feel satisfied and to turn down the drive to fill your plate. The natural sugar in fruits, called fructose, also has an appetite-reducing effect.

What this means is that if you have included generous amounts of rice, potatoes, beans, fruits, and other carbohydrate-rich foods on your meals, the calories in pork chops, salad oil, and other fattening foods are less likely to find their way onto your fork.

How do you get these "negative calorie effects?" You will not get them from steak or fried chicken, because there is virtually no complex carbohydrate in fish, chicken, beef, milk, eggs, or any other animal product. Complex carbohydrates are found only in plants. Grains, vegetables, and beans are loaded with them. That is why vegetarian foods are such powerful foods for permanent weight control.

If you like, you can forget technical terms like carbohydrate. As long as your diet is made from grains, beans, vegetables, and fruits, rather than animal products, it will be naturally rich in carbohydrate.

20 Foods You Can Eat
in Virtually Unlimited Portions

Listed below are 20 foods that you should feel free to eat in very generaous portions. Unless you are really stuffing yourself, you can eat as much of these as you want. In fact, there are many more than 20, as you have learned. One caveat: Enjoy these with no butter, margarine or oily toppings—fats are fattening!

Corn	Celery
Rice	Peas
Potatoes	Cauliflower
Lettuce (all varieties)	Pineapple
Broccoli	Cabbage
Carrots	Oranges
Black beans	Apples
Kidney beans	Grapefruit
Spinach	Bananas
Lentils	Oatmeal

Cutting Out Fats and Oils

Now for the most important part of the food prescription:

✦ Cut out the fats and oils.
✦ Fats and oils are packed with calories.
✦ Fat in foods is fat on you.

These are the most calorie-dense part of the foods we eat. As we noted previously, every single gram of fat or oil holds nine calories. This is true for all fats and oils: beef fat, chicken fat, fish oil, vegetable oil, and any other kind of fat or oil.

In the May 1991 issue of the *American Journal of Clinical Nutrition*, researchers at Cornell University published the results of a fascinating experiment. They had kept volunteers on different diets for several weeks. They found that those who ate foods that were very low in fat and high in carbohydrates lost weight steadily, *without limiting how much they ate*. But those on high-fat diets could not effectively lose weight even if they ate skimpy portions. A similar phenomenon was found by Dr. T. Colin Campbell of the China Health Study, a massive and on-going research undertaking.[6] His team found that Chinese populations eat a very high carbohydrate diet with enormous quantities of rice. They eat very little in the way of animal products, and so, get little fat in their diets. Overall, their diets contain more calories than most Americans eat, but they stay much slimmer, both because of the very low fat content and high carbohydrate content of the diet, and because they stay physically active, which we will discuss later. The first key to emphasize is the need to shift from fatty foods to carbohydrates.

There are various kinds of fat. The main categories discussed by dietitians are *saturated fat,* which is common in animal products and is solid at room temperature, and *unsaturated fat,* which is common in vegetable oils and is liquid at room temperature. Different kinds of fat have different effects on your cholesterol level. But:

✦ For weight control, we need to be concerned about all forms of fat.

✦ All fats and oils have the same calorie content: 9 calories in every gram.

About 40 percent of the calories most Americans get every day come from fat. For a typical 2000-calorie menu, that is 800 calories each day just from fats and oils in our foods. By cutting out most of the fats in our diet, we can cut out hundreds of calories. To put it another way, if all the foods we eat are very low in fat, we can eat far more food than we could on a high-fat diet, without more calories.

We should cut our fat intake from 40 percent of the calories we eat down to about 15 percent. Eating 15 percent of our calories from fat is a substantial reduction. It is a powerful weight-reducing step and yields other tremendous benefits as well. We must go on a "search and destroy" mission for fat. *Be on the look out for fat in the two forms in which it comes: animal fat and vegetable oil.*

Look out for ALL fats!

Animal fat was designed by nature to act as a calorie-storage area for animals. When you eat animal fat, you are eating all those stored calories. Animal fat is not only on the outside of a cut of meat. It is marbled through the lean part, too, almost like a sponge holding water. So, if you are eating meat you are eating someone else's fat and someone else's concentrated stored calories. It will put fat on you. Let's take some examples:

Imagine that we are making tacos. Let's compare two recipes for taco filling, one made with ground beef and the other with beans. Beef is high in fat; three ounces of ground beef hold about 225 calories. Beans are very low in fat, and three ounces hold only about 80 calories. So we can cut out nearly two-thirds of the calorie content by switching from the beef recipe to the bean recipe. A big part of the difference is the very high fat content of the ground beef and the very low fat content of beans. About 60 percent of the calories in ground

Food	Percentage calories from fat
Potato	less than 1 %
Peas	3 %
Black beans	4 %
Macaroni noodles	4 %
Vegetarian baked beans	4 %
Rice	less than 5 %
Cauliflower	6 %
Spinach	7 %
Broccoli	8 %
Wheat bread	15 %
Whole milk	49 %
2% milk	35 %
Extra lean gound beef	54 %
Ground beef	60 %

beef come from fat. This is a huge load of calories that do nothing good for the body and do a lot of harm, from promoting heart disease to increasing cancer risk, and, of course, fattening you up.

Take a look at the fat content of various foods in the chart on the previous page. Remember, the fat contents listed here are percentages of calories, not percentages by weight. This is a critical difference. Whole milk, for example, is 3.3 percent fat

Whole Milk

3.3% Fat By Weight

49% Fat By Percent of Calories

2% Milk

2% Fat By Weight

35% Fat By Percent of Calories

by weight, because it is loaded with water. But 49 percent of its calories come from fat. Milk that is two percent fat by weight is actually about 35 percent fat as a percentage of calories. It is actually not a low-fat product at all.

"Extra lean" ground beef is really not so lean either: it derives 54 percent of its calories from fat. It is an abysmal food for people concerned about their waistlines. Even McDonald's McLean DeLuxe burger is not a low-fat food. Although the company advertises it as "91 percent fat-free," they are using the weight percentage, not the calorie percentage. By calories, the McLean DeLuxe patty is 49 percent fat, hardly something anyone would recommend.

By calorie content, here's a listing of common meat cuts:

Common Meat Cuts

Cut	Percentage of calories from fat
Chuck roast	51 %
Rib eye steak	63 %
Short loin porterhouse	64 %
Hotdogs	82 %
Bologna	83 %
Most beans, grains, vegetables	less than 10 %

Even the beef industry in its "lean" advertisments of the "skinniest six" beef specimens could not find any cuts of meat that are anywhere near the fat content of beans, grains, or vegetables:

"Skinniest Six" Meat Cuts

Cut	Percentage of calories from fat
Tenderloin	41 %
Top loin	40 %
Sirloin	38 %
Round tip	36 %
Eye of round	32 %
Top round	29 %
Most beans, grains, vegetables	less than 10 %

All of these have many times the fat content of typical vegetables, beans, grains, and fruits.

The problem with meats, including poultry and fish, is that they are muscles, and muscles are made up of protein and fat. They contain no fiber at all and virtually no carbohydrate.

Advertisers sometimes claim that chicken and fish are low-fat foods. Are they? Let's look at the worst and the best of the poultry line:

Poultry	Percentage of calories from fat
Chicken frank	68 %
Roasted chicken	51 %
White meat w/out skin	23 %
Most beans, grains, vegetables	less than 10 %

The chicken also contributes about 85 mg. of cholesterol. In addition, chicken pushes carbohydrates and fiber off your plate. No matter how chicken is prepared, it cannot get its calorie level down to that of the truly healthful foods, because chicken, like all meats, is permeated by fat and contains no complex carbohydrates or fiber. *Fat always has more calories than carbohydrate.*

Some people eat fish in the hope that fish oil will reduce their cholesterol levels. Actually, fish oils reduce triglycerides but do not reduce cholesterol levels. And it should be remembered that fish oils are as fattening as any other oils or fats. Like all fats and oils, they contain nine calories per gram.

Different types of fish differ greatly in their fat content:

Fish	Percentage of calories from fat
Chinook salmon	52 %
Atlantic salmon	40 %
Swordfish	30 %
Halibut	19 %
Snapper	12 %
Sole	9 %
Haddock	8 %

Many of these are as bad as other animal products. Others are in the same ballpark as vegetables as far as their fat content goes, but this does not make them recommended foods. Remember fish contains no complex carbohydrates and no fiber, and tends to displace these foods from the meal. All fish products also contain cholesterol and far too much protein, (see pages 41-44) in addition to contamination problems. So, fish is still not a health food, although certain types of fish are much lower in fat than are beef and poultry.

In summary, meats, poultry, and fish have two main problems for those concerned about their weight:

First, like all muscles, they have inherent fat, adding concentrated calories.

Second, because muscle tissues are mainly just protein and fat, they reduce the carbohydrate and fiber content of the diet. They displace the fiber and carbohydrates that are essential to a satisfying and metabolism-boosting menu.

✦

The first prescription for cutting the fat is the V-word:
vegetarian foods are power foods
for weight control.

The second issue is vegetable oil.

✦

Vegetable oils have received a good reputation because they contain no cholesterol and are low in saturated fats. But their calorie content is the same as any other kind of fat. That should be emphasized. *All fats and all oils, regardless of type (lard, pork fat, chicken fat, olive oil, fish oil, etc.), are packed with calories: nine calories per gram.* They are all the enemies of those in search of a slimmer waistline.

Let's take an example with vegetable oils: As you know, a potato is a low-fat food that is also modest in calories. Only about one percent of the calories in a potato come from fat.

When the potato is baked or prepared as mashed potatoes, no extra oil is added. But if the potato is cut into french fries and dropped in cooking oil, its fat content soars up to 40 percent or more. As a result, its calorie content doubles or even triples.

Compare the fat content of a doughnut (50 %), which is fried in oil, to a bagel (8 %), which is not. The doughnut has more than six times the fat of the bagel.

Fat in foods adds easily to your fat stores.

1 Large Raw Potato			2 Regular Fries
70 Calories	+	Frying =	440 Calories
.1 gram fat			23 grams fat

Little or no conversion is needed in the body before the fat we eat passes through the digestive tract and the blood stream to the fat tissues of the body. But the energy in carbohydrates cannot be easily stored as fat. The body has to do a considerable amount of work before those calories can be stored, and many calories are lost in the process.

Fats Are Calorie-Dense	
Carbohydrate	4 calories per gram
Protein	4 calories per gram
Fat	**9 calories per gram**

Fat and Other Health Considerations

There are other serious problems with fats, too. Fat in foods contributes substantially to the risk of several forms of cancer (breast, colon, prostate, and others), heart disease, diabetes, gallstones, and numerous other problems as well. Although animal fats are the worst, vegetable oils also increase health problems.

A low-fat menu is a recipe for a slim, healthy body. It can take some getting used to because, unfortunately, people crave high-fat foods. Grease is like an addicting substance. We all have a tendency to return to fried chicken, greasy burgers, potato chips, and fried onion rings, so be on the look-out. It is easier to cut them out entirely than to continually tease oneself with occasional greasy foods.

Getting Free from the Fat in Foods

As you know from the above discussion, shifting away from fat and toward high-fiber foods means getting away from animal products. Cutting out animal products can greatly reduce your fat consumption. Avoiding added vegetable oils and fried foods is another very powerful step. Here are some suggestions on how to do it:

Salad Dressings: Salad dressings can be packed with fat. A salad made of one cup of romaine lettuce with half a tomato holds only 20 calories. But look what adding a tablespoon of dressing will do:

Salad dressing (1 Tbsp.)	Fat content
Catalina french dressing	5.5 grams of fat (65 calories)
vinegar and oil (50/50 mix)	8 grams of fat (72 calories)
Good Seasons Zesty Italian	9.2 grams of fat (85 calories)

So the salad with dressing has four to five times the calories of a salad without dressing.

Low-fat or no-fat dressings cut down substantially on the fat content. Look at the brands that are now available at the grocery store, often in the "dietetic section." Or you might prefer a sprinkle of lemon or lime juice as a dressing for salad or vegetables. A tablespoon of lemon or lime juice has no fat and only four calories. You may also find that you enjoy the taste of fresh spinach, chick peas, tomatoes, or other salad ingredients with no dressing at all.

Baked Goods: In recent years, nutritionists have made distinctions between saturated (animal fat, tropical, and hydrogenated oils) and unsaturated (most vegetable) oils, because the former contribute to heart problems. But if our goal is to slim down, the issue is much simpler: all kinds of fats and oils are problems. They are all packed with calories. Some baked goods, such as bagels, pretzels, and many breads, are usually quite low in fat. On the other hand, croissants, cakes, pies, and cookies tend to be very high in fat. Commercially packaged goods list their ingredients on the label. The ingredients are listed in decreasing order of their quantities, so if oil is one of the first ingredients, there is probably more of it than if it is one of the last listed ingredients. In addition, most labels provide enough information to allow you to calculate the actual fat content, using the simple formula on the next page (page 36).

We do need some fat in the diet. But we need only a fraction of what most of us typically get. A small amount of fat is inherent in grains, legumes, and vegetables. This is all the body needs. Children can (and perhaps should) have a bit more fat in their diet. Breast milk is naturally higher in fat for the needs of growing infants. The natural process of weaning eliminates this nutrient when it is no longer appropriate.

How To Check The Fat Content Of Foods

How much fat is in foods we eat?

What is important is the percentage of calories that comes from fat. (The percentage of fat by weight is not important, because it can be easily thrown off by the water content of products.)

Some manufacturers are starting to list the percentage figure, but, if they do not, it is still easy to calculate. On the information panel on the package, notice the number of grams of fat in one serving. Multiply by nine (every gram of fat contains nine calories). Then divide by the number of calories per serving. Then multiply by 100.

$$\frac{\text{grams of fat} \times 9}{\text{calories in serving}} \times 100 = \% \text{ calories from fat}$$

Let's try an example. Here is an information label from a supposedly low-calorie pizza:

NUTRITIONAL INFORMATION
Serving size ... 1.0 oz   Carbohydrates ... 7.2 g
Servings per pkg ... 8   Fat ... 2.5 g
Calories ... 65   Sodium ... 74 mg
Protein ... 3.1 g   Cholesterol ... 1 mg

This serving is incredibly small, so all the numbers will be artificially low. But even so, the key to look for is the percentage of calories that come from fat. One serving contains 2.5 grams of fat. If we multiply by nine and divide by the number of calories per serving (65), we come out with .35. Then multiplying by 100 gives us 35 percent. This means that 35 percent of the calories in this product are from fat. This is better than fried chicken or a hot dog, but still higher than we want. Not such a healthful entree after all.

$$\frac{2.5 \times 9}{65} = .35 \times 100 = 35\% \text{ of calories from fat}$$

Reggie:
Swearing Off Grease

Reggie called himself a 'grease addict.' Potato chips, French fries, buttered popcorn, peanuts, peanut butter, and onion rings were all part of his routine. He had been fairly slim until he reached about 25 when his waistline gradually began to expand. Now, at 40, he is about 20 pounds overweight. His daily intake of fatty foods had a predictable effect.

He did not plan to give up any foods totally. But as an experiment, he decided that for three weeks he would eat only low-fat vegetarian meals. From a set of recipes, he made bean entrees with lots of vegetables on the side. There was no limit on amounts, but he was very strict to omit all oils, margarine, salad dressings, and all meats and dairy products. After three weeks, he had lost about three pounds. That was not a big drop, but he found that he had lost all desire for greasy foods, and now associated them with his weight problems. So he decided to stick with his new way of eating for three more weeks. He lost five more pounds. A month later, he had lost another 5 pounds. He now weighs the same as he did in college.

His friend Morris adopted the same program. He weighed 275 pounds when he started. Without limiting calories, he lost 80 pounds. His girlfriend used the same method to drop from 150 to 120 pounds.

Fat Substitutes

Chemical fat substitutes have recently emerged in the news. *Simplesse*, made by the NutraSweet Company, is made of a protein that simulates the texture of grease on the tongue. Because it changes consistency when heated, Simplesse can only be used in foods which are not baked or fried. *Olestra* is a sucrose polyester made by Procter and Gamble. It is designed to taste and feel like fat, but is indigestible and unabsorbable. Its safety is a matter of vigorous dispute; some contend that Olestra causes cancer and liver problems.

I find it impossible to be enthusiastic about these products. Like chemical sweeteners, their safety remains in doubt. In addition, they reinforce the taste for fat, rather than helping you to get away from the taste for grease.

To reduce the fat content of the diet, low-fat vegetarian foods are ideal. Vegetarian foods are obviously free of the animal fat that permeates meats, poultry, and fish. Steering clear of fried foods and added oils is the other half of the equation. Spaghetti with tomato sauce, bean burritos, vegetable curries, baked potatoes, and salads are a few examples of foods that can be very low in fat, yet delicious.

Check Your Knowledge

Let's review. For each pair below, see if you can pick which is lower in fat. You'll find the answers below. Do not skip this part. It is easy, but important.

Which is lower in fat?
1. Fried chicken vs. broiled top round beef
2. Leanest beef vs. leanest chicken
3. Leanest chicken vs. vegetarian baked beans
4. Leanest beef vs. rice
5. Leanest chicken vs. potato
6. Spaghetti with tomato sauce vs. a Lean Cuisine spaghetti with meatballs dinner
7. Spaghetti with meat sauce vs. spaghetti with tomato sauce
8. Fast-food meat taco vs. fast-food bean burrito
9. Cheddar cheese vs. bread
10. Peanut butter vs. rice
11. Ice cream vs. jelly beans
12. Baked potato vs. french fries
13. Doughnut vs. bagel

Answers
(The numbers given are percentages of calories from fat):
1. Broiled top round beef (38 %) is lower in fat than fried chicken (50 % fat), but both are high-fat foods.
2. The leanest chicken is about 20 % fat, and lower than the leanest beef (29 % fat), although both are high in fat compared to grains, beans, vegetables, and fruits.
3. Vegetarian baked beans (4 % fat) are much lower in fat than even the very leanest chicken (20 %).
4. Rice (0.8 %) is much lower in fat than the leanest beef (29 % fat).
5. A potato (1 %) is much lower in fat than the leanest chicken (20 % fat).

39

6. Spaghetti with tomato sauce (6 %) is much lower in fat than a Lean Cuisine spaghetti with meatballs dinner (23 %).
7. Spaghetti with tomato sauce (6 %) is lower in fat than spaghetti with meat sauce (35 %).
8. A fast-food bean burrito (31 %) is lower in fat than a fast-food meat taco (50 %). A home-made burrito can be much lower in fat.
9. Bread (16 %) is much lower in fat than cheddar cheese (74 %). Most cheeses are extremely high in fat.
10. Rice (0.8 %) is much lower in fat than peanut butter (78 %).
11. Jelly beans (0.8 %) are much lower in fat than ice cream (48 %), although both hold a very large amount of sugar.
12. A baked potato (1 %) is much lower in fat than french fries (47 %).
13. A bagel (8 %) is much lower in fat than a doughnut (50 %).

Carbohydrate-rich foods are vital for long-term weight control. Take the carbohydrate test below:

Which has more carbohydrate?
1. A fish fillet vs. broccoli
2. Bread vs. beef
3. Milk vs. potato
4. Cheese vs. rice

Answers:
(The numbers given are percentages of calories from carbohydrate):
1. Broccoli is 78 % carbohydrate. A fish fillet has no carbohydrate at all.
2. Bread is 75 % carbohydrate. Beef has no carbohydrate at all.
3. A potato is 93 % carbohydrate. Milk is 30 % carbohydrate, in the form of simple sugar.
4. Rice has much more carbohydrate (89 %) than cheese (1 %).

What About Protein?

Protein is the subject of many myths. The bottom line on protein is this: High-protein diets are dangerous. Many formula diets emphasize high-protein foods and contain very little carbohydrate. This type of diet is not a formula for success. It can cause a rapid, and usually temporary, water loss. But usually the weight comes back on very quickly.

In addition, there are serious dangers to high-protein diets: osteoporosis and kidney disease. The bone-thinning disease of osteoporosis is an epidemic in the U.S., and protein has apparently been a big part of the cause. High-protein diets cause calcium to be lost in the urine. This has been shown repeatedly in scientific studies. When subjects consume foods that are overly high in protein, especially animal protein, they excrete calcium. For example, if volunteers were to eat meals with a substantial meat content and later have their urine tested, calcium would often be found in the urine. Since Americans tend to eat meat daily, it is likely that they are routinely excreting calcium. The calcium does not come from the meat. It comes from their bones.

There are several theories that scientists have used to explain this. The amino acids which make up protein and are released when protein is digested make the blood slightly acidic. In the process of buffering this acid, calcium is pulled from the bones. Ultimately it is discarded in the urine. In addition, meat protein is very high in what are called "sulfur-containing amino acids." These are suspected of being particularly likely to leach calcium from the bones.

While many of us grew up being taught to make sure we got enough protein, the fact is we have gotten too much. Our bodies only need a fraction of what we generally get. When we eat two or three times the amount of protein the body can use, much of it is broken down and excreted. In the process, it not only interferes with the calcium balance of the body, it can also overwork the kidneys. The excess of amino acids acts as a diuretic, increasing the flow of urine. The amino acids eventually break down to urea, which acts as a diuretic, too. The overall effect is to force the kidneys to work much harder than they should. The nephrons, which are the kidneys' filter units, gradually die off in the process.

We need protein in the diet, but we do not need a large overdose of protein. The problems of calcium loss and kidney damage occur, not just in those who consume high-protein formulas, but in people who consume meat, chicken, or fish on a regular basis.

The best advice about protein is to stick with plant sources. A varied menu of grains, beans, and vegetables contains more than enough protein for human needs. There is no need to carefully combine proteins. Any variety of plant foods provides sufficient protein. When meats are included, the protein content easily becomes more than the body can handle safely. For example, if you were to have a single seven-ounce serving of roast beef, you would get 62 grams of protein. This one serving contains more than the recommended daily allowance of protein for a whole day (a range of 44-56 gms., depending on your age and level of activity), unless you are pregnant or nursing.

Let's take a look at two other high-protein products, egg

whites and skim milk. Doctors learned long ago that egg yolks were loaded with cholesterol. A single egg yolk contains 213 mg. of cholesterol (and is 80 % fat). That is even more cholesterol than in an eight-ounce steak. But while many doctors now recommend avoiding egg yolks, some still encourage the consumption of egg whites because they contain protein. Well, the fact is that egg whites contain *too much* protein. Of the calories in an egg white, fully 85 % are from protein. That is a huge amount that no one needs. (In addition, salmonella bacteria are an increasing problem in eggs, even those with intact shells.)

Skim milk is a similar wrong turn. Because of the high saturated fat content of whole milk, many people have chosen skim dairy products. Getting rid of the dairy fat is certainly a good idea, because the fat in whole milk, butter, cheese, cream, and ice cream will tend to increase cholesterol levels and elevate cancer risk. But after the fat is removed, skim milk is hardly a health food. It contains no fiber, and no complex carbohydrates, but has a substantial amount of lactose sugar (55 % of calories). Antibiotics are also frequently present in milk products, due to their routine use on farms.

If you thought you needed milk for strong bones, you have been the victim of an extremely aggressive advertising program by the dairy industry which was not based on good science. The fact is that people in countries which consume milk routinely tend to have weaker bones than those in

Protein Myths

1. Milk for strong bones
2. Egg whites are good
3. Vegetarians do not get enough protein.

countries which avoid milk. Osteoporosis is more likely due to excess protein in the diet and to sedentary living. It is not due to a "milk deficiency," and milk consumption does not slow the osteoprosis that commonly occurs in older women.

There are also concerns about the *type* of protein in milk. Milk proteins often cause allergies and other health problems. There are indications that milk proteins contribute to juvenile-onset diabetes, and specialized cow proteins (antibodies) are now known to cause colic in infants. Like it or not, nature designed cow's milk for baby cows, not for people.

Limit Alcohol

In general, health recommendations have been mixed on alcohol: Modest alcohol consumption—one to two drinks per day—does not promote heart problems. On the other hand, even small amounts of alcohol increase the risk of breast cancer and contribute to birth defects. And, of course, beyond modest use, alcohol contributes to many other very serious health problems, from accidents to heart disease, cancer, neurological disorders, and digestive problems.

What about its effect on your waistline? This is no mystery. Alcohol is fattening. People who consume beer, wine, or mixed drinks on a regular basis get a big load of extra calories, as this list shows:

Drink	Calories
Wine (4 oz.)	85
Light Beer (12 oz.)	100
Beer (12 oz.)	150
Liquor (1.5 oz.)	124
100 proof gin, rum, vodka or whiskey	

These figures are not presented for you to remember, but rather to illustrate that the alcohol in these beverages packs a significant number of calories.

What is important about alcohol, however, is not just its calorie content. The important point is this: *Alcohol adds to the calories you are already consuming, rather than displacing any*. For example, if you were to eat four bread sticks before dinner, you would eat a bit less at dinner. The 150 calories in the bread would displace about the same amount from the food you would have later. But alcohol does not seem to have this same sort of compensatory mechanism.[3] If you substitute a beer for the bread sticks, it also holds 150 calories, and the calories from alcohol are not compensated for by eating less later. The calories in alcohol *add* to what you eat.

The presumption is that although soft drinks hold about the same number of calories as beer (a can of cola holds about 155 calories), they are much more likely to be compensated for later than are the calories in alcoholic beverages, since the calories in soft drinks come from sugar. For mixed drinks, the calories in the drink mix are not so likely to contribute to your girth as the calories in the alcohol which is added to it. This is not a recommendation for colas and drink mixes. The point is that alcohol can really widen your waistline. For alcoholics, the effects are different. Alcoholics often consume less food than do non-alcoholics and are deficient in a host of nutrients.

Sweets and Sweeteners

Concentrated sugars, such as hard candies, are just chunks of simple sugars and lack any fiber or water. As a result, they are as concentrated a form of calories as can be found in a carbohydrate food. If you consume large quantities of sugary foods, such as sweets and sodas, you will get more calories than the body needs.

But even so, sugars are not nearly as calorie-dense as fats. If you are not controlling the amount of fat you are eating, there is little point in worrying about sugar.

Often, sugar is not the main problem in sweets. In cookies, pies, and cakes, there may be a lot of sugar, but there is usually a huge amount of fat, too.

Sweets	Percentage of calories from fat
Haagen-Dazs ice cream	57 %
Hershey dark chocolate bar	50 %
Chips Ahoy cookies	42 %
Pillsbury German Chocolate cake	40 %

When selecting sweet foods, pick those with the lowest amount of fat. How about fruit for dessert? And sodas should be replaced with spritzers or water.

Forget artificial sweeteners. They are no answer to weight problems. First of all, they do not seem to have much power to help in weight control. Using an artificial sweetener instead of a teaspoon of sugar saves you only 16 calories. But just two grams of fat hold more calories than the teaspoon of sugar. That is not to say that you should consume sugar, but it is to say that artificial sweeteners are a distraction from the real dietary issues, which for most people relate to the fat content of the diet.

More importantly, artificial sweeteners are poisonous. We have seen this over and over again. Cyclamates can cause cancer. The same may be true of saccharin, although it remains on the market with warning labels on each package. Aspartame, marketed under the name NutraSweet, has problems of its own. Substantial evidence links aspartame to a variety of effects on the brain. Headaches are common, and there is currently a scientific debate over whether aspartame can cause grand mal seizures and whether children, including babies developing in the womb, may suffer brain damage if exposed to aspartame. I see no value in chemical sweeteners.

Check Your Knowledge

Try each question. Do not skip any. Answers are listed below.

1. How do alcoholic beverages affect weight problems?
2. What problems are caused by diets with too much protein?
3. Is there a lot of fat in pies and cookies?
4. True or false: As far as protein is concerned, the more the better.
5. True or false: Vegetarians get enough protein without carefully combining foods.

Answers:

1. Alcohol contains calories, and we do not compensate for this by eating less later.
2. Osteoporosis and kidney problems.
3. Yes.
4. False. We need some protein, and the amount in plant foods is sufficient. Adding high-protein products is not healthful.
5. True.

Watch Out For Stuffing

Most overweight people do not overeat. Most actually eat less than thin people do. But some people do overeat. For one of many reasons, they are "stuffers;" they keep eating long after others would have had enough. It is important to identify whether you are a member of that minority of overweight people who do tend to overeat so you can learn what to do about it. Let's look at three principal reasons for overeating:

1. *The Restrained-Eater Phenomenon:* As we saw earlier, one big reason for an episode of overeating is the restrained-eater phenomenon, which kicks in after periods of very-low-calorie dieting. This can affect anyone, even people who have never had a tendency to binge or to overeat for any psychological reason. The key, of course, is to avoid the very-low-calorie regimens that tend to produce binges.

2. *Eating in Response to Emotions:* Ask yourself these questions:

✦ Is food your usual answer to stress?
✦ Do you eat when you are not at all hungry?
✦ Do you eat throughout the day?

If the answer to any of these is yes, then this section may be for you.

Some people eat when they are under stress. Depression, anxiety, hurt feelings, anger, or sadness are answered with a trip to the kitchen. This is easy to identify, and a bit harder to remedy. Do not expect to plumb the depths of your psyche and rearrange its contents in short order. For now, you need to make a plan to compensate for this tendency.

Anticipate that from time to time, like it or not, you will become angry or sad or frustrated with things, and plan to deal with these feelings in another way. Is there someone you can talk to, or someone you can call? If food is serving as a comfort, what other comforts can you take advantage of? For example, are there certain places, photographs, books, or clothes that serve as comforts, too?

Deal with emotions in ways that are inconsistent with eating. For example, if you plan to get together with a friend, be with someone who is not preoccupied with eating, and pick a place where eating will not occur—meet in a park or office instead of a restaurant. Then as mealtime approaches, fill up on healthful foods first.

Some people may use overweight as a defense. A heavy body may fend off intimacy or other anxiety-provoking encounters. The vast majority of overweight people are not in this category, but, if you are, it will be helpful to recognize it.

Are you eating out of boredom? We need many forms of nourishment: friends, intellectual challenges, physical activities, romance, challenges and successes in our lives, rest, and sleep. When these are absent, food may become a cheap substitute. Is food taking the place of something else?

If you are saying, "I overeat, but I do it because food tastes so good," it may be worth examining what else occupies your time. If your life is filled with boredom, then food may well be the most exciting thing in it. It is important to see what prevents you from engaging more fully in other activities that make life what it is.

I would like to refer you to two additional resources. First, Overeaters Anonymous has helped many, many people. Their number is listed in your telephone book. If you really are overeating, OA can be a terrific help. Second, there is a book by Victoria Moran, called *The Love-Powered Diet,** which is entirely devoted to helping people who eat in response to emotions. It has more helpful information on dealing with overeating than any other book I have seen.

3. *Carbohydrate Craving:* There is a group of people who have a particular craving for carbohydrates. It is not because of their taste; the foods can be either sweet or starchy. It is apparently due to an effect carbohydrates have on brain chemistry. Carbohydrates boost a brain chemical called serotonin, which is important in brain functions, including sleep and mood regulation. Most antidepressants increase serotonin levels in the brain, among other actions. One theory is that carbohydrate cravers have naturally low levels of serotonin and, so, tend to be depressed. They eat large quantities of carbohydrates because they have noticed that it helps them to feel better.

That is the theory. Here is the chemistry behind it: Carbohydrates break down in the body to sugars, which, in turn, stimulate insulin secretion. Insulin is a hormone produced in the pancreas. It helps get sugar out of the blood stream and into the cells of the body. Now that is not all insulin does. It also helps amino acids, which are the building blocks of protein, to get out of the blood stream and into the cells. So, after a carbohydrate-rich meal, insulin drives the sugar and the amino acids out of the blood and into the cells.

Now here is the interesting part: As the insulin drives the amino acids out of the blood, it leaves behind one particular amino acid called tryptophan. Tryptophan stays behind because it is stuck to a large carrier molecule. Without all the other amino acids around, tryptophan has less competition for getting into the brain. So the tryptophan passes into the brain, where it is converted to serotonin, which can alter moods, and cause sleepiness.

---

*New World Library/Publishers' Group West, 1992

Carbohydrates Can Aid Sleep
By Increasing Tryptophan In The Brain

The bottom line is that carbohydrate-rich meals increase serotonin in the brain. Carbohydrate cravers tend to become depressed in the winter months when the days are short. Food may help normalize their brain chemistry.

There is nothing wrong with a high-carbohydrate menu. As we have seen, carbohydrates are very important. The key is to select foods rich in complex carbohydrates, such as rice and other grains, beans, and vegetables, rather than sugar candies or sugar-fat mixtures which really will add to one's waistline.

The Role of Physical Activity

Our lives have become all too sedentary. We have eliminated most of the physical activities that got our blood moving when we were younger and that kept our ancestors fit. It is terrific to bring physical activity back into our lives, for four reasons:

1st Movement burns calories
> Every movement you make, whether it is blinking your eyes or lifting a grand piano, burns some calories. The more we move, the more calories we burn.

2nd Regular physical activity boosts your metabolism.
> Calories are burned more quickly, not only while you are exercising but also afterward for a period of time.

3rd Physical activity helps preserve your muscle mass
> Muscle tissue has a rapid metabolism and is much better than fat tissue at burning off the calories we ingest. If your muscles waste away from inactivity, your body burns fewer calories per hour.

4th Physical activity helps control the appetite
> Twenty minutes of exercise before dinner reduces the appetite slightly. This seems to be particularly true for activities that warm the body, such as tennis, running, or dancing (Some people experience an *increase* in appetite after cooling exercises, such as swimming.) Unfortunately, it is likely that overweight people experience less (or even none) of the exercise-induced change in appetite than do normal-weight individuals, so this may be a mechanism that helps people stay thin rather than helping people to get thin.[4]

There are numerous other benefits of physical activity, from reduced risk of heart disease and cancer to more energy and a more relaxed outlook on life. You may find that you will sleep more soundly when your body is tired from exercise. In turn, better sleep makes you feel like taking care of yourself. Chronically tired people prop themselves up with all sorts of indulgences, including unhealthful foods, that do not seem so important when they are well rested.

How Much Activity?

Let's start with a half-hour walk every day, or, if you prefer, an hour three times per week. Pick a place to walk that is enjoyable for you. Enjoy the sights, sounds, and smells.

Feel free to substitute any equivalent activity in place of walking. Here are some examples of physical activities and the number of calories they burn:

Activity	Calories
A brisk half-hour walk:	120
A leisurely half-hour bicycle ride:	140
A half-hour ping-pong game:	210
A half-hour swim:	240
A half-hour jog:	284
An hour of gardening:	300
An hour of golf:	356
An hour of tennis:	456

The key is to have fun. Choose something you'll enjoy.

If you like dancing, gardening, bike-riding, a run with your dog, or a vigorous walk in the woods, then off you go! Bring a friend along if you can. Making activity a social event decreases the possibility of drifting back into sedentary living. At work, use the stairs instead of the elevator.

If you have access to a health club, you will find all sorts of sports and physical activities that turn exercise into pleasure. The old gym has really been transformed into an environment that makes physical activity fun and tailors it to the individual.

Start slowly, particularly if you have been sedentary for some time. If you are over 40 or have any history of illness or joint problems, talk over your plans with your doctor. And remember, stick with activities that you really enjoy.

If you have been on a low-calorie diet, you should switch to a low-fat, high-carbohydrate menu without calorie restriction before you begin any program of regular vigorous exercise. The reason is that the low-calorie diet probably slowed down your metabolism. Even though exercise will boost the metabolic rate of most people, it can actually have the opposite effect on people who have been starving themselves. So stop the calorie restriction first, then, after a couple of weeks, add physical activity.

What About Genetics?

There is one factor we cannot control, and that is our genetic inheritance. Like it or not, if your parents were both thin, you and your siblings will tend to be thin. If your parents were heavy, you will have a similar tendency.

We also tend to inherit our parents' shape. If your parents were apple-shaped, carrying their weight in their chests and abdomens, you are likely to be apple-shaped as well. If they were "pears," carrying their weight in their hips and thighs, you are likely to be pear-shaped as well. There are all sorts of shape variations. Size is more easily changed than shape. If you carry your weight in your hips, as you lose weight you might become a skinny "pear," but you will still be a "pear."

Fat on the abdomen is easier to lose than hip fat. Although hip fat is more difficult to remove, it is also less likely to contribute to health problems. To determine whether you are at greater risk of health problems from being overweight, take a tape measure and measure around your waist and around your hips. For men, increased risk of health problems begins when your waist is bigger than your hips. For women, they begin when your waist is more than 80 percent of your hip measurement.

If you have passed that point, your weight problem is not a cosmetic issue anymore. It is a very real contributor to heart problems, cancer, diabetes, and a broad range of other problems that you do not want to have.

Some people believe that, because there is a strong genetic component to our size and shape, there is nothing they can do to lose weight. This is not true. Although the genetic factors that are passed from parents to children exert important effects, we do not just give our children DNA. We also give them recipes. We give them attitudes about food and preferences for various kinds of food. We also tend to pass along an interest or disinterest in physical activity, and attitudes about health and about how our bodies should look. These can all be modified, if we decide to do so. Whatever hand we have been dealt by our inheritance, there are still steps we can take to change our weight.

The key about genetics is to remember that it is only one of several factors that affect your weight. It shows your tendency. But within that tendency, there is a great deal that you can do to help reach the body size you want.

A Word About B12

Vitamin B12 is needed in minute amounts for healthy blood and healthy nerves. It is not made by plants or animals; it is made by microorganisms, such as bacteria and algae. In traditional societies, B12 is produced by bacteria found in the soil and on vegetables. It also can occur naturally in the process of preparation of foods, such as Asian miso or tempeh, soyfoods which are loaded with the vitamin. In the West, modern hygiene and pasteurization have eliminated these traditional sources. Meat-eaters get the vitamin B12 that bacteria produce in the digestive tracts of animals and passes into the animals' tissues, but people who adhere to a vegetarian diet (as I recommend) should pick up a supplement.

All common multivitamins (One-A-Day, Flintstones, StressTabs, etc.) contain B12. The RDA for B12 is only two micrograms per day. Health food stores carry vegetarian vitamin brands which are free of dairy and meat extracts. Your body has a very good supply

of this vitamin already, but if you have been on a strict vegetarian diet for three years, you should begin taking at least 3 micrograms per day of any common supplement of vitamin B12.

Summary of Basic Concepts

Let's summarize the major points:

Diet: The overall dietary changes are simple.

✦ Eat foods from plant sources: grains, beans, vegetables, and fruits.

✦ Avoid animal products

✦ Keep vegetable oil to a minimum as well.

What these simple steps do is to cut way down on fat, reduce protein content moderately, and give us the metabolic boost of carbohydrates, plus lots of fiber.

✦ Avoid calorie restrictions.

Unless you are really stuffing yourself, you can enjoy unlimited quantities of foods. If you really are overeating, you will need to address the psychological factors that prevent you from treating your body better.

✦ Refined sugars and alcohol should be avoided as well.

It is not necessary to resolve to change your eating habits for the rest of your life. All you can change is what you are doing today. And tomorrow, you can make the same decision again, if you like. But you do not need to plan what you will eat 20 years from now. I point this out because sometimes the idea of life-long change can be frightening. Don't worry about it. *All you need to work on is what you are doing today. And if you like it, you can stick with it.*

To get the results you want, do not water down these guidelines. Adding occasional servings of chicken or french fries will erode your progress. Give yourself the best.

Physical Activity:

✦ Walk for a half-hour per day or an hour three times a week.

Or substitute any equivalent activity. Have fun. The cumulative effect can be enormous.

Part II

Let's Get Started

Let's Get Started

A Step-by-Setp Program

In Part I, we learned the basic concepts. Now it's time to put them into action by tasting new foods, trying new food stores, activating our muscles, and making a solid change in our lives.

Adapting to a new, improved menu is surprisingly easy. It does take a little time, about three to six weeks for a new habit to become routine, but soon you will wonder why you did not try this before.

First, give yourself a pat on the back. You wanted a change for the better, and here you are, well on your way there. You've already covered a lot of ground in learning about slimming down. Now we will put knowledge into practice. Here is how we will proceed:

1st We will throw out all the high-fat foods that have caused so many problems for us.

2nd We will bring in new and interesting foods that are powerful for permanent weight control.

3rd We will set up a simple, effective program of physical activity that will help burn off the pounds.

Planning for Success

One reason this program works is that it provides a very powerful food program, linked with physical activity. But it does more: it takes into account what human beings need in order to make a major change in eating habits.

Let's face it: it's not always easy to change habits. *But certain things make it much easier and much more likely to stick.*

I recently reviewed several major research projects in which people were asked to change their diets. In some of these projects, the participants changed their diets very dramatically, and in others they hardly changed at all. It became very clear that the programs which yielded the most changes were those which had certain things going for them. These factors have been incorporated in this program:

1. *Asking for the degree of change you want.* Doctors or researchers who sell their patients short with weak recommendations get nothing more than they ask for.
2. *Don't just read about foods; taste them as well.* That will be a major focus of this chapter.
3. *Go for maximal reward.* Nothing is more encouraging than success. So this program not only uses foods, it also brings in enjoyable physical activity designed for what people want most: permanent weight control.
4. *Simplicity in foods.* This program is designed to be easy to remember, with no need for charts, measuring, or limiting serving sizes. The two rules of thumb are:

➔Use no animal products.
➔Keep vegetable oils to an absolute minimum.

These simple guidelines are extremely powerful for long-term weight control.

5. *Foods must be enjoyable.* That means quality and quantity. So this program will use tasty foods and no calorie restriction.
6. *Change completely.* Do not tease yourself with foods. Anyone who has tried to change a habit knows about this one. Let's take smoking as an example. If people try only to cut down on smoking, they get essentially nowhere, because the taste for tobacco is always fresh in their minds. It is very easy to increase the frequency of a habit that has not yet been broken. But if they quit completely, they can get some distance between themselves and tobacco and can start a new habit—the habit of being a non-smoker. The same is true of foods. If you have fried chicken or potato chips once a week, then you are constantly teasing yourself with the taste of these very fattening products. If, however, you get away from these foods completely, you allow a new habit to start; you are getting the force of habit working with you, starting a new habit.
7. *Think short-term.* There is no need to make any resolution about what you will do in the distant future. All you can control is what you are doing now. So plan to follow this program for three weeks. At the end of that time, see how you feel. Notice its effect on your waistline. And if you like what you see, you can try it again for another 21 days. If you continue, you will get its full benefit. If you stop, you will lose all your gains. But think short-term; do not burden yourself with feeling the need to make resolutions for the distant future.
8. *Family and friends.* Our families eat with us. They eat the food we prepare or, perhaps, prepare the food we eat. Having them on our side is a terrific boost. When researchers have worked with patients to modify their diets, they have found that including the family makes a tremendous amount of difference. So ask them to join you in this program. Now, they may not feel a need for

any permanent change in their eating habits. And you do not need to ask them to change permanently. All you need to ask them is to join you while you are working on this program. In many cases, they will want to read it with you. That is the ideal. They will benefit from this program, too. This new way of eating not only slims waistlines; it can also lower cholesterol levels, help control blood pressure, help prevent cancer, and prevent many conditions from constipation to varicose veins. At the very least, however, your family and friends must not tempt you with unhealthful foods while you are working through these lessons, and you must not prepare any unhealthful foods for them.

Frequently families get stuck in old habits. They may even want to talk you out of changing and may forecast failure. In that case, you need to have a short sit-down talk. Tell them that if they care about you, they will understand that this is very important to you. They will help and not hinder you. If you have done this with sufficient sincerity, they will be overcome with guilt and will plead for forgiveness. (You might suggest that they can make it up to you by doing your shopping for you.)

Get them to think of it as a three week adventure in eating, including foods from a host of exotic foreign locales. Involve your kids in the kitchen, learning about new foods by helping you prepare them. My previous book, *The Power of Your Plate*, was written for skeptical family members, and you may wish to give a copy to them. For those who do not enjoy reading, a new cassette tape, *Live Longer, Live Better* is also available.

Follow this program to the letter. **Do not "cheat."** You are embarking on a powerful and rewarding program. Give it every chance for maximal success. You deserve no less, and I believe you will be really pleased with the results.

Getting Offending Foods
Out of the House

The first step is to throw out the foods that have been problems in the past and which will get in your way in the future. You can throw them away or give them away, but the key is to get them completely out of the house.

Before you begin, have a meal. It is very difficult for a hungry person to throw any food product away, no matter how unhealthful it may be. Then go on a search and destroy mission for the high-fat, no-fiber foods in your house. Get rid of all of the following:

Any meat, poultry, or fish products
All dairy products, including butter, milk or cream,
                yogurt and cheese.
Margarine
Vegetable oil. (Yes even olive oil.)
All salad dressings other than non-fat dressings
Cookies, cakes, pies and ice cream, other than non-fat
Potato chips
Nuts and nut butters
Sugary candies

You may notice a certain sense of relief as you rid yourself of these unhealthful products. Now we will stock our shelves with foods that will help us have the body we want.

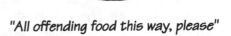

"All offending food this way, please"

Getting to Know New Foods

We are going to go shopping for new kinds of foods and will learn how to prepare them. Don't worry, they are all easy to fix. Our goal for right now is not to be gourmet cooks, but to learn new kinds of foods and to adapt our tastes to a lower-fat menu. If you like, gourmet recipes can come later.

The foods listed on the following pages create a simple beginning menu, but they are important for you to get to know. They are powerful for slimming down. Some are already quite familiar; others may be new. Some will seem very humble, but do not be deceived. They taste terrific and also have an excellent combination of nutritional factors that make them among the most powerful foods for keeping pounds off permanently.

Eat before shopping!

The emphasis in this list is on convenience and simplicity, with minimal preparation time. For example, you will see canned beans, rather than dried beans. Later, you may wish to cook from scratch, instead of using canned varieties. Frozen vegetables are also included for convenience. Their nutritional value is generally good, and better than canned vegetables.

We will start with a one-week menu. The idea is to stock your kitchen with enough healthful foods to give you a good start on adapting to new food tastes. It will also eliminate the need for frequent shopping trips, which are times of vulnerability to unhealthful impulse purchases.

Most of these items are available from any grocery store, but a few are found only at health food stores, as I will indicate. Notice that you do not have to mix any diet powders, and you certainly do not have to go hungry.

Do not go shopping on an empty stomach. If you do, you risk ending up buying anchovy-packed olives and coconut cream pie and avocado swirl-cake and all the other impulse purchases that seduce hungry stomachs.

People with food allergies should obviously skip any food to which they are allergic. If you are on a sodium-restricted diet, look for low-sodium varieties of canned foods, or compensate with less sodium in other foods. Health food stores often stock low-sodium products.

People on prescribed diets should follow this program in consultation with their health care professional. For example, because these foods improve insulin's efficacy, diabetics may need to reduce their insulin use. Similarly, people with high blood pressure may find they need less of their medication as well. Persons with high triglycerides may need to limit fruit.

Keep in touch with your
health care professional

First, let's take a look at the foods we will be starting with. Then I will give you a shopping list you can use to guide your trip to the store.

Breakfast

1. **Fresh fruit:** Melon, grapefruit, oranges, bananas, pineapple, or any other fruit you like. It can be your entire breakfast, or just the beginning.
2. **Hot cereal:** Choose from old-fashioned rolled oats, grits, or other hot cereal. Cooked versions are best, but instant is acceptable. If you like, top with cinnamon, or try strawberries, raisins, or other fresh fruit. Do not use milk.
3. **Whole-grain toast.** Have plain, or top with jelly or cinnamon. Do not use butter, margarine, or cream cheese.
4. **Cold cereal with soymilk.** Choose whole-grain cereals. Soymilk is not only free of animal fats; it is also free of the cholesterol and lactose that are found in dairy products. Use only low-fat soymilk, such as Edensoy or Westbrae Lite vanilla flavor (soy milk is carried at any health food store, or in regular groceries near the condensed milks).
5. **Black beans on toast.** This Latin American breakfast sounds unusual, but can be popular on both sides of the border. Simply empty a can of black beans into a saucepan and heat. Spoon the beans onto toast and top with a touch of mild salsa or Dijon mustard. One can of black beans holds two generous servings.
6. **Chick peas (garbanzo beans).** Open a can of chick peas and rinse. Eat plain or with non-fat salad dressing. One can holds two generous servings.

(If you are like me, you will be surprised to see these last two. But try them! You're in for a treat.)

Lunch

At lunch time, convenience is often a key. Low-fat lunches not only help you slim down, they also prevent the after-lunch fatigue that follows high-fat meals.

1. ***Instant soups.*** Health food stores stock a wonderful variety of split pea soup, couscous, noodle soups, and others. These are easy to keep in your desk at work, since you just add hot water. (If you prefer, bring a thermos of vegetable or split pea soup from home.)

2. ***Bread, bread sticks, pretzels, Melba toast.***

3. ***"Finger vegetables"***: cherry tomatoes, baby carrots, broccoli & cauliflower tops with non-fat dressing.

4. ***Fresh fruit***: Enjoy bananas, apples, pears, oranges, etc., as well as fruit like kiwi and fresh pineapple for a change of pace. Avoid avocados.

5. ***Sandwich:*** Have a CLT: Cucumber, lettuce, and tomato, on whole-grain bread. Add onion and mustard, if you like. Some people like to add sprouts. Unfortunately, most traditional sandwich fillings are loaded with fat. Avoid meats of any kind, cheese, mayonnaise, and peanut butter.

6. ***Chick peas.*** It's easy to keep a can of chick peas in a desk drawer at work. Simply rinse and serve plain, or with non-fat salad dressing.

7. ***Leftovers from dinner or breakfast*** are always welcome. Microwave if you like.

8. ***If you eat lunch in a cafeteria,*** enjoy the cooked vegetables, potatoes, or the salad bar, using a twist of lemon juice instead of dressing. Avoid all meats, eggs, dairy products, and keep vegetable oils to an absolute minimum.

Dinners

In planning meals, I suggest starting with vegetables, usually including two different ones at each meal. Then, add a grain or other starch, such as rice, potatoes, or pasta. Include a bean dish and finish with a serving of fruit. Be generous with grains and other starches, and have smaller portions of bean dishes.

1. ***Vegetables.*** Try broccoli, spinach, carrots, cauliflower, green beans, peas, lima beans, Brussels sprouts, kale, asparagus, succotash, or any other. Any fresh vegetable is fine: spinach leaves, carrots, celery, Boston lettuce or other greens, plus any other salad vegetables that strike your fancy: peppers, tomatoes, cauliflower, etc. If you like, top vegetables with a sprinkle of lemon or lime juice, minced garlic, onion, or parsley. Avoid butter or margarine, sour cream, and other fatty toppings. Do not use oil as a topping or for sautéing or frying. Frozen vegetables are convenient and similar in nutritional value to fresh vegetables. Choose plain varieties, not those in cream sauce.

2. ***Grains and other starches:***
   a. Rice is one of the best foods for slimming down. It is very low in calories and very nutritious. At the grocery store, notice the variety of boxed rice dishes, such as curried rice, long grain and wild rice, brown rice, pecan rice, basmati rice, risotto with tomato, or rice pilaf. Nearby, you will see the fabulous mixes for couscous, tabouli, and vegetarian burgers. Avoid any mixes with meat products or a high fat content. At the health food store, you will find organic short-grain rice, which is an excellent choice (see recipe on page 156). Or try any other varieties of rice that catch your fancy.
   b. Spaghetti with tomato sauce. Whole-grain spaghetti is best. If you are stuck with regular spaghetti,

consider it acceptable for now, even though much of its fiber has been removed. Of commercial tomato sauces, choose those lowest in fat.

c. Bread. Whole-grain varieties are always best.

d. Corn. Corn is a grain, not a vegetable. Enjoy the natural taste of corn without butter, margarine, or oil.

e. Potatoes. Baked, mashed (instant is fine), steamed or boiled. No hash browns, potato chips, or french fries. If you like, a dab of Dijon mustard or ketchup is okay. If you like gravy on potatoes, pick up a can of Franco American Mushroom-Flavor Gravy. Do not add milk to mashed potatoes, and use no butter, sour cream, margarine, cheese, or other fatty toppings.

3. *Legumes (beans, peas, and lentils):*

a. Black beans. Do not skip this one. Black beans are a delightful discovery. They are extremely low in fat, packed with fiber, and delicious. Top with mild salsa or mustard. If you are new to black beans, I strongly suggest buying them canned (note that different brands vary widely in their sodium content), rather than cooking up dried beans, which requires considerably more time. In case you were worrying, for most people, black beans do not seem to cause much gassiness.

b. Vegetarian baked beans. Several canned varieties are available at grocery stores, and are very convenient.

c. Lentil soup. Progresso and other companies make delicious, low-fat lentil soups. For those on sodium-restrictions, health-food stores carry low-sodium varieties.

4. *Fruits.* Pears, cherries, strawberries, peaches, apples, bananas, pineapples and just about any other fruit make great desserts or garnishes for other foods.

Part III

Moving Into High Gear

Moving Into High Gear

A Step-by-Step Program

Now you have dramatically cut the fat content of your diet, and boosted the carbohydrate and fiber content. This encourages a steady and permanent weight loss, which is improved with exercise. In effect, if your fat stores were a huge bag of water, you just poked a small hole in it. Slowly and surely it will drain out.

In this chapter we will move beyond the simple meals we discussed in Part II, and have a look at how to bring an essentially limitless variety of foods and new food ideas into your life. We will also deal with some of the pitfalls that can sometimes get in our way.

New Recipes, New Foods

First, let's open the doors to new kinds of foods. The variety of healthful foods is enormous, thanks to the many countries that have had culinary traditions very different from our own and to the ever-growing interest in nutrition.

Eating Out

When choosing restaurants, the best ones for low-fat, vegetarian foods are Chinese, Japanese, and other Asian cuisines, Middle-eastern, Indian, Mexican, and Italian. Traveling is a time of challenges to those trying to eat in a healthful way, but many fast-food restaurants have responded to the demand with baked potatoes and salad bars. Taco restaurants feature bean burritos, and the turnpikes of the East Coast even feature spaghetti restaurants in their travel plazas. In your car, bring some fresh fruit or sandwiches along. When you book a flight request a vegetarian meal or fruit plate; all airlines now have them.

Collecting New Recipes

The next time you get a chance, browse through the cookbook section of your local bookstore. There is an astounding wealth of new cookbooks, particularly those offering vegetarian cuisine. They are a goldmine of food ideas. Look at the wonderful pastas, Middle-eastern foods, Asian foods, and on and on. Some use dairy products or more than minimal amounts of oil, but these recipes can often be modified, as noted on page 84. If you have not already seen my earlier book, *The Power of Your Plate*, I would strongly recommend it as a source of in-depth information on a broad range of nutrition issues, as well as many of my own favorite recipes.

New Food Products

Exploring new food products can be delightful as well. Take a look at the health food store. There is a wonderful range of new products, from soups of every variety, dips, and sandwich fillings to exotic entrees that are a snap to prepare. New brands of tortilla chips are baked rather than fried and, so, are oil-free. Many varieties of rice and other grains produced without chemical treatments are there. Delightful beverages are now available ranging from flavored waters to juices and teas.

There is also a huge range of non-meat "transition foods"—foods that take the place of ice cream, mayonnaise, hot dogs, hamburgers, and most other fatty, cholesterol-packed foods. These substitutes are not always good for everyday use, however. While better than the items they imitate, they are often still rather high in fat.

Resource Groups

If there is a vegetarian society in your area, get in touch with them. They have been exploring healthful eating for years, and can be a great source of information.

Tune Up Your Menu

In the last chapter, we brought high-fiber, high-carbohydrate foods to the center of the plate. Now, let's fine-tune things a bit:

Whole grains:

Let whole grains (as opposed to processed grains) play a greater role in your diet. "Processed" grains are ground (e.g. flour) or have some of the fiber removed (e.g. white rice). Evidence indicates that whole grains release a bit fewer of their calories. So rice, rolled oats, or corn may release even fewer calories than flour made from whole grains. Let rice replace bread.

Raw foods:

Be increasingly generous with raw vegetables and fruits. Many people report remarkable weight reductions when they include large amounts of raw fruits and vegetables in their diets. This is partly because these foods are extremely low in fat and high in fiber and carbohydrate, but there may be other contributors that science has not yet unraveled. People with even stubborn weight problems have benefited greatly by eating more raw vegetables and fruits.

When you select raw vegetables, skip the iceberg lettuce; it's mostly water. For a salad, try fresh spinach and the other delightful greens in the produce department. Add peppers, broccoli, celery, carrots, cauliflower, cooked chickpeas, or whatever else you might like. Happily, it is now easier to find vegetables produced without pesticides.

Again, skip dressings that include oil. Enjoy the taste of vegetables without added flavorings.

Modifying recipes:

Recipes that are high in fat can often be easily modified to lower fat content. You will note that often the amounts of oil added to recipes are quite arbitrary. Once you have "re-set" your taste for fat, you will automatically want to leave the grease out of the foods you prepare.

Health food stores sell egg replacer that does exactly that, drastically cutting down the fat content of baked goods. An egg-sized piece of tofu will also accomplish much the same thing in a baking recipe. TVP (texturized vegetable protein), a de-fatted soy product sold at health food stores, replaces ground beef so well that many pizza companies and other ground beef users have already made the switch.

For fat-free frying:

If you are sautéing in oil, here's a helpful tip: Let's say your recipe for spaghetti sauce calls for sautéing onions and garlic in olive oil. How many calories are there in three tablespoons of olive oil? Would you believe 360? Instead, try this: put a half-cup of water in a sauce pan and sauté your onions and garlic in simmering water. You get no extra calories and a pleasant, lighter taste.

The new non-stick pans work remarkably well with this method.

Activity and Rest

Increase physical activity naturally. If you are comfortable with your current level of physical activity, let the time you give it increase naturally. Do not force it, or it will become a chore. But let yourself enjoy an extra night out dancing or bowling, a day on the golf course, or walking in the park. The keys, again, are *fun* and *frequency.*

Get plenty of sleep. People need rest. Chronically tired people have no energy to exercise. Often they feel so out of sorts that they are tempted to prop up their flagging spirits with food or alcohol. There is no substitute for adequate sleep.

Troubleshooting

If you have had insufficient results so far, be patient; slow weight loss is more likely to be permanent than rapid weight loss.

But if you did not lose weight at all, then let's review the basics:

- ✦ Were you using any oily foods, such as salad dressings, peanut butter, or margarine?
- ✦ Are you buying fatty products, such as tofu hotdogs?
- ✦ Were there any animal products in your foods?
- ✦ How about alcohol?
- ✦ Did you miss out on regular physical activity?

If you had problems in any of these areas, now is the time to address the problem squarely. There are always solutions to these problems, and tremendous rewards when you do.

Are you having trouble sticking to healthful foods with friends? It may be that you are looking to others for approval, and afraid that they will not sympathize with your new and healthful way of eating. If so, I have noticed a remarkable thing in the past few years. Every time the subject of vegetarian foods comes up in conversation, or I ask a waiter for a vegetarian entree, such as a vegetable plate or spaghetti when there was not one on the menu, I always find that they already know that this is a very healthful way to eat. Many are already vegetarians themselves, or at least recognize that they should be. So stop worrying.

When eating out with friends, suggest Italian, Chinese, or Mexican restaurants. At American-style restaurants, do not hesitate to ask for a vegetable plate. The National Restaurant Association asked all its members in 1991 to feature vegetarian entrees, because, at that time, about one in five diners looked for them. If you don't see it on the menu, by all means ask.

When I am invited to a party, I always say something along the lines of "I am a vegetarian, and I don't want to put you to any trouble. How about if I bring along something like a meatless spaghetti sauce or hummus?" Invariably, my offer is declined, because they planned to have a meatless dish or two. Often, they say that their son or husband is a vegetarian, and it is no problem at all.

Some people have digestive troubles. Any major change in diet can be a temporary challenge for the digestive tract. A meat-eater who becomes a vegetarian suddenly has to adapt to a high-fiber diet. If a vegetarian were to become a meat-eater, a similar problem would occur due to the enormous change in the dietary contents. Any change can lead to temporary indigestion or gas. If this happens to you, be aware that the effect is a temporary price you are paying for your past indiscretions.

Some plant foods—certain varieties of beans, in particular—do tend to cause gas. Try to pin down which is the problem food. Pinto beans, for example, may be a problem, while black beans are not. Include more grains in the diet, such as rice, and deemphasize beans. A new product, called Beano, is sold at health food stores and is reported to eliminate the gassy effect of foods.

Good Luck!

This program is so elegantly simple, yet it is the most effective way to control your weight permanently. The great part is that there is no need to count calories, skip meals, or eat small portions. You can enjoy food in reasonable quantities, and enjoy it in a slimmer, healthier body.

I hope you will let me know how this program works for you. Please write to me at the Physicians Committee for Responsible Medicine. PCRM can also keep you posted on the latest in nutrition through our magazine, *Good Medicine*.

Let me wish you the very best of health and success in your new venture.

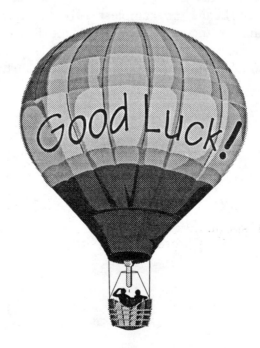

References

[1] Foster GD, et al. Controlled trial of the metabolic effects of a very-low-calorie diet: short-and long-term effects. Am J Clin Nutr 1990;51:167-72.

[2] Danforth E, Jr., Sims EAH, Horton ES, Goldman RF. Correlation of serum triiodothyrone concentrations (T3) with dietary composition, gain in wight ad thermogenesis in man. Diabetes 1975;24:406.

[3] Spaulding SW, Chopra IJ, Sherwin RS, Lyall SS. Effect of caloric restriction and dietary composition on serum T3 and reverse T3 in man. J Clin Endocrinol Metab 1976;42:197-200.

[4] Mathieson RA, Walberg JL, Gwazauskas FC, Hinkle DE, Gregg JM. The effect of varying carbohydrate content of a very-low-caloric diet on resting metabolic rate and thyroid hormones. Metabolism 1986;35:394-8.

[5] Welle S, Lilavivathana U, Campbell RG. Increased plasma norepine concentrations and metabolic rates following glucose ingestion in man. Metabolism 1980;29:806-9.

[6] Chen J, Campbell TC, Junyao L, Peto R. Diet, lifestyle, and mortality in China. 1990, Oxford University Press, Oxford.

[7] de Castro JM, Orozco S. Moderate alcohol intake and spontaneous eating patterns of humans: evidence of unregulated supplementation. Am J Clin Nutr 1990;52:246-253.

[8] Kissileff HR, Pi-Sunyer FX, Segal K, Meltzer S, Foelsch PA. Acute effects of exercise on food intake in obese and nonobese women. Am J Clin Nutr 1990;52:240-5.

Part IV

Menus and Recipes

Easy Ways to Cut the Fat

- Get the animal products out of your diet. Meat, dairy products, and eggs are major contributors of fat.
- Grill and oven-roast foods instead of frying them.
- Select baked versions of fried foods, like baked tortilla chips, potato chips, and pretzels.
- Avoid deep-fried foods like doughnuts; have a bagel instead.
- Use nonstick pots and pans, which allow food to be prepared with little or no added fat.
- "Saute" in liquid instead of in fat:
    Heat ½ cup of liquid (water, vegetable stock wine, dry sherry) in a large pot or skillet. Add the vegetables to be sauteed and cook over medium-high heat, stirring occasionally, until the vegetables are tender.
- When it is absolutely necessary to saute or fry in oil, nonstick vegetable oil sprays allow you to do so with a fraction of the fat.
- Use a microwave oven to reheat foods.
- Use fat-free dressings on salads.
- Seasoned rice vinegar and balsamic vinegar are great for dressing salads.
- Eat cooked vegetables plain, or with a sprinkling of seasoned rice vinegar or lemon juice.
- Try your favorite fat-free salad dressing on cooked vegetables.
- Replace the oil in salad dressing recipes with seasoned rice vinegar, vegetable stock, bean cooking liquid, or with water.
- Use the cornstarch and water mixture below to

thicken salad dressing:

Whisk 1 tablespoon of cornstarch with 1 cup water. Heat in a small saucepan, stirring constantly, until thick and clear. Refrigerate. Use in place of oil in any salad dressing recipe. May be kept refrigerated for up to three weeks.

. Make soup thick and creamy by adding a cooked, mashed potato or instant mashed potato flakes.

. Limit your consumption of avocados, nuts and seeds, and coconut, which are all high in fat.

. Replace ice cream with fruit sorbet or a frozen fruit smoothie.

. The amount of fat in baked goods can often be reduced without affecting the taste or texture of the finished product.

. Experiment with your recipes: start by reducing the fat by half. You may have to add a bit of extra liquid to achieve the desired consistency.

. Applesauce, mashed banana, prune puree, or canned pumpkin may be substituted for the fat in many baked goods.

A Few Ingredients
That May Be New to You

Most of the ingredients in the recipes are commonly available in grocery stores. A few which may be unfamiliar are described below.

Basmati rice is a flavorful variety of long-grain rice sold in natural food stores and many supermarkets. Brown basmati rice is less refined than white basmati rice.

Bulgur is toasted, cracked wheat which cooks quickly and has a delicious, nutty flavor. It is sold in natural food stores and often in supermarkets as "Ala".

Couscous is made from wheat that is cracked rather than ground. It is sold in the grain section of many supermarkets, natural food stores, and ethnic markets. Whole wheat varieties are found in some natural food stores.

Diced chilies are mild chilies (like Anaheim) which are available canned or fresh. "Ortega" is a widely-sold brand. If you use fresh chilies, remove the skin by charring it under a broiler then rubbing it off.

Nutritional yeast adds flavor and nutritional value to foods, and is a rich source of B vitamins (look for brands which include vitamin B-12). It is similar to "brewer's yeast," but better tasting. You'll find it in natural food stores.

Red pepper flakes are dried, crushed chili peppers sold in the Mexican food or spice section of many supermarkets.

Reduced-fat tofu is found in natural food stores and many supermarkets. Also try silken tofu, a smooth, delicate variety that is excellent for sauces, cream soups, and dips. One popular brand, Mori-Nu, is available in most grocery stores.

Rice milk is a mild-flavored beverage made from rice. Delicious on cereal and as replacement for cow's milk in most recipes. Available in natural food stores and a growing number of supermarkets.

Roasted red bell peppers add great flavor and color to a dishes. Roast your own or purchase them already roasted, packed in water, in most grocery stores.

Soy milk has none of the cholesterol or animal fat of cow's milk. It comes in a variety of flavors, as well as in low-fat and vitamin- and mineral-fortified versions. Soymilks vary widely in flavor, so try several to find the ones you like best. Available in natural food stores and in many supermarkets.

Swanson's Vegetable Broth is a widely available and very convenient canned broth.

Tahini is sesame seed butter used in Middle Eastern cooking. It is available in natural food stores and many supermarkets.

Textured vegetable protein (TVP) is an excellent meat substitute for sauces, chili, and stews. It is easy to use and is available in natural food stores.

Unbleached flour is white flour that has not been chemically whitened. Available in most grocery stores.

Balsamic vinegaris a delightful and mellow-flavored wine vinegar available in most grocery stores.

Seasoned rice vinegar is flavored with a bit of sugar and salt and is great for salad dressings and on cooked vegetables. Available in most grocery stores.

Whole wheat pastry flour is milled from soft spring wheat. It retains the bran and germ and, at the same time, produces lighter-textured baked goods than regular whole wheat flour. Available in natural food stores.

Seven Days of Great Meals

Day One

Breakfast   Orange Julius (page 99)
             Whole Grain Toast
             Unsweetened Fruit Preserves

Lunch   Spanish Rice (page 135)
             Quick Black Bean Chili (page 160)
             South of the Border Salad (page 119)

Dinner   Sweet & Sour Vegetable Stirfry (page 150)
             Brown Rice (page 132)
             Steamed Kale (page 142)
             Peach Cobbler (page 167)

Day Two

Breakfast   Whole Wheat Corncakes (page 101)
             Fresh Fruit Slices

Lunch   Mixed Greens Salad (page 118)
             Balsamic Vinaigrette (page 115)
             Potato and Corn Chowder (page 125)
             Whole Grain Bread

Dinner   Broccoli Burritos (page 158)
             Bulgur (page 136)
             South of the Border Salad (page 119)
             Melon slices

Day Three

Breakfast   Cinnamon Orange French Toast (page 104)
                 Maple Syrup
                 Fresh fruit

Lunch   Tomato Soup (page 124)
                 Mixed Greens Salad (page 118)
                 Piquant Dressing (page 115)
                 Whole Grain Bread

Dinner   Pita Wedges with Hummus (page 113)
                 Curried Mushrooms with Chickpeas
                        (page 165)
                 Couscous (page 137)
                 Steamed Kale (page 142)
                 Dried Figs

Day Four

Breakfast   Quick Breakfast Rice (page 107)
                 Fresh Fruit Smoothie (page 100)

Lunch   Ensalada de Frijoles (page 123)
                 Warm Corn Tortillas

Dinner   Polenta with Hearty Barbecue Sauce
                        (page 149)
                 Mixed Greens Salad (page 118) with
                        Piquant Dressing (page 115)
                 Potatoes with Kale and Corn (page 143)
                 Chocolate Torte (page 168)

Day Five

Breakfast   Fruit & Bagel Breakfast (page 105)
             Fresh Fruit Smoothie (page 100)

Lunch   Hoppin' John Salad (page 122)
             Curried Sweet Potato Soup (page 130)
             Whole Grain Bread

Dinner   Thai Vegetables with Rice (page 152)
             Braised Cabbage (page 141)
             Ginger Peachy Bread Pudding (page 166)

Day Six

Breakfast   Blueberry Muffins (page 109)
             Hot Cereal
             Fresh Fruit

Lunch   Golden Mushroom Soup (page 126)
             Cucumbers with Creamy Dill Dressing
                (page 117)
             Garlic Bread (page 111)

Dinner   Vegetarian Burger (page 155)
             Potato Salad (page 120)
             Corn on the cob
             Watermelon

Day Seven

Breakfast   Cinnamon Apple Oatmeal (page 106)
             Fresh Peach Smoothie (page 100)

Lunch   Minestrone (page 127)
             Three Bean Salad (page 121)
             Garlic Bread (page 111)

Dinner   Chili Mac (page 154)
             Mixed Greens Salad (page 118)
             Balsamic Vinaigrette (page 115)
             French bread
             Banana Freeze (page 170)

Stocking Your Pantry
for Healthful Eating

By keeping some basic foods on hand, you can prepare quick, nutritious meals at a moment's notice. Some of the items listed below are ingredients which show up frequently in recipes.

Others are healthful, quick choices for those days when there just isn't time to cook. If you were to take an inventory of my pantry, here is what you would find (brand names for some items are shown in parentheses):

Dry Goods

cold breakfast cereals without added fat or
    sugars
hot breakfast cereals
eggless pasta: fettuccine, spirals, lasagne, etc.
brown basmati rice
white basmati rice
quick cooking brown rice (Lundberg)
bulgur wheat
couscous
polenta
rolled oats
whole wheat flour
whole wheat pastry flour
unbleached flour
cornmeal
popcorn
dried lentils
split peas
pinto beans
raisins

instant soups: vegetarian soup cups, ramen
soups
black bean flakes (Taste Adventure, Fantastic
Foods)
pinto bean flakes (Taste Adventure, Fantastic
Foods)
reduced-fat silken tofu (Mori Nu)
vegetable broth: powder, cubes, or canned
vegetable oil spray
baking soda
baking powder

Canned foods (canned goods should be used within one year)

canned beans, including kidney, garbanzo,
black, pinto, etc.
canned tomatoes, tomato sauce, tomato paste
canned pumpkin
applesauce
vegetarian soups (made without fat)
vegetarian baked beans (Bush's, Heinz)
vegetarian chili beans (Dennison's, Health
Valley)
fat-free refried beans (Rosarita, Old El Paso,
Bearitos)
vegetarian spaghetti sauce (make without fat)
salsa

Breads

whole grain bread (may be frozen)
flour tortillas (may be frozen)
corn tortillas (may be frozen)

Produce

pre-washed salad mix
pre-washed spinach

broccoli
kale or collard greens
yellow onions
garlic
red potatoes
russet potatoes
yams or sweet potatoes
winter squash
green cabbage
carrots
celery
apples
oranges
bananas

Frozen foods (should be used within 6 months)

apple juice concentrate
orange juice concentrate
frozen corn
frozen peas
frozen bananas
frozen berries
frozen chopped onions
frozen diced bell peppers
fat-free vegetarian hot dogs (Smart Dogs, Yves
    Veggie Wieners)
fat-free vegetarian burgers (Garden Vegan, Boca
    Burger, Natural
Touch Burger by Morningstar Farms)

Seasonings and Condiments

herbs and spices: cinnamon, ginger, cloves,
    ground cumin,
cayenne, chili powder, red pepper flakes, curry
    powder, basil,

oregano, black pepper
low-sodium soy sauce
fat-free salad dressing (Good Seasons makes an
    excellent dry mix)
seasoned rice vinegar
balsamic vinegar
cider vinegar
stone ground mustard
ketchup
unsweetened fruit preserves
molasses
maple syrup
sugar
salt

BREAKFAST FOODS

Orange Julius

Makes 2 1-cup servings

If you ever enjoyed an Orange Julius at a shopping mall or the county fair you're in for a real treat, because this one is as good for you as it tastes. It's quick to make too, if you keep frozen bananas on hand. Just peel the bananas, break them into chunks, and pack them loosely in an airtight container to freeze. They will keep well for about 3 months.

> **1 large orange, peeled**
> **¼ cup vanilla soy milk or rice milk**
> **¼ cup oat bran**
> **1 teaspoon sugar**
> **½ teaspoon vanilla**
> **1½ cups frozen banana chunks**

Combine all ingredients in a blender and process on high speed until completely smooth and thick.

Per 1 cup serving: 170 calories; 4 g protein; 35 g carbohydrate;
1 g fat; 13 mg sodium; 0 mg cholesterol

Fresh Fruit Smoothie

Makes 2 servings

Start your day out right with this delicious and satisfying beverage.

  1 large orange, peeled
  1 cup frozen banana chunks
  1 cup frozen strawberries
  ½ cup apple juice

Combine all ingredients in a blender and process on high speed until completely smooth.

Per 1 cup serving: 134 calories; 2 g protein; 30 g carbohydrate;
0 g fat; 6 mg sodium; 0 mg cholesterol

Fresh Peach Smoothie

1 serving

This smoothie is so thick and rich it's actually like a frozen dessert. Keep frozen bananas on hand so you can whip it up any time.

  1 fresh ripe peach (or nectarine)
  1 frozen banana (about 1 cup banana chunks)
  ½ cup vanilla soy milk

Combine all the ingredients in a blender and process on high until completely smooth.

Per serving: 187 calories; 4 g protein; 40 g carbohydrate; 1 g fat;
46 mg sodium; 0 mg cholesterol

Whole Wheat Corncakes

Makes 16 3-inch pancakes

Serve these nutritious pancakes with fresh fruit, fruit preserves, or maple syrup.

    ½ cup whole wheat flour
    ½ cup cornmeal
    ½ teaspoon baking powder
    ¼ teaspoon baking soda
    ¼ teaspoon salt (optional)
    1 small ripe banana, mashed
    2 tablespoons brown sugar
    1 tablespoon vinegar
    1-1¼ cups soy milk or rice milk

Stir the flour, cornmeal, baking powder, baking soda, and salt together in a mixing bowl.

In a separate bowl, combine mashed banana, brown sugar, vinegar and 1 cup of soy milk or rice milk. Add to the flour mixture and stir just enough to remove lumps and make a pourable batter. Add a bit more milk if the mixture seems too thick.

Preheat a nonstick skillet or griddle. Spray lightly with a vegetable oil spray. Pour small amounts of batter onto the heated surface and cook until the tops bubble. Turn with a spatula and cook the second side until golden brown, about 1 minute. Serve immediately.

Per pancake: 44 calories; 1 g protein; 9 g carbohydrate; 0 g fat;
65 mg sodium; 0 mg cholesterol

Buckwheat Pancakes

Makes about 20 3-inch pancakes

These pancakes are made with yeast, which makes them light and tender without added fat. Start the batter about 1½ hours before you want to serve the pancakes, since it needs an hour to rise.

> 1 cup buckwheat flour
> ½ cup unbleached or whole wheat pastry flour
> ½ package active dry yeast (1½ teaspoons)
> ½ teaspoon salt (optional)
> 1¼ cups very warm water (about 100° F)
> ½ teaspoon baking soda
> 1 tablespoon molasses
> ¼ cup very warm water (about 100° F)

Preheat the oven to 200° F, then turn it off. In a large bowl, mix the buckwheat and unbleached flours, the yeast, and salt.

Stir in 1¼ cups of warm water and beat until smooth. Cover the bowl with a plate and place it into the preheated oven to rise until very bubbly, about 1 hour (Be sure the oven is turned off!).

Dissolve the soda and molasses in ¼ cup of very warm water and add it to the buckwheat batter. Heat a nonstick skillet or griddle. Mist it lightly with vegetable oil spray. Pour small amounts of batter onto the heated surface and cook until puffed and bubbly. Turn and cook the second side about 1 minute. Serve immediately with syrup, fruit preserves, or fresh fruit.

Per pancake: 31 calories; 1 g protein; 6 g carbohydrate; 0 g fat;
75 mg sodium; 0 mg cholesterol

Sourdough Waffles

Makes 8 5-inch waffles

Sourdough starter can be used to make delicious, light waffles any added fat or cholesterol. Specialty food stores sell sourdough starter mixes, or better yet, get some from a friend who keeps sourdough starter. The care and feeding of sourdough is really quite simple. Simply use it every two weeks and replenish it with equal amounts of flour and water.

1 teaspoon baking soda
2 tablespoons maple syrup
2 cups sourdough starter

Combine the soda and maple syrup in a mixing bowl and stir to mix. Add the sourdough starter and mix well.

Cook the batter in a preheated, oil-sprayed waffle iron until golden brown, 3 to 5 minutes. Serve immediately.

Per waffle (without oil): 58 calories; 2 g protein; 13 g carbohydrate;
0 g fat; 103 mg sodium; 0 mg cholesterol

Cinnamon Orange French Toast

Makes 4-6 slices

French toast is quick to prepare, low-fat, and cholesterol-free when you make it without eggs. Vary the bread you use for different flavors and textures (cinnamon raisin is my favorite).

> **1 cup soy milk or rice milk**
> **3 tablespoons cornstarch**
> **1 tablespoon orange juice concentrate**
> **1 tablespoon maple syrup**
> **1 teaspoon vanilla**
> **½ teaspoon cinnamon**
> **⅛ teaspoon salt**
> **4-6 slices whole grain bread**

Mix the soy milk or rice milk, cornstarch, orange juice concentrate, maple syrup, vanilla, cinnamon, and salt. Pour the mixture into a broad, flat dish. Coat each slice of bread on both sides with the mixture.

Preheat a nonstick skillet or griddle and mist it with a vegetable oil spray. Add the bread slices and cook until the first side is golden brown, about three minutes. Turn carefully with a spatula and cook the second side until golden brown, about 3 minutes. Serve hot with maple syrup or fruit preserves.

Per slice: 119 calories; 3 g protein; 24 g carbohydrate; 1 g fat;
143 mg sodium; 0 mg cholesterol

Fresh Fruit & Bagel Breakfast

Serves 1

Enjoy a bagel and fresh fruit for a quick and satisfying breakfast or snack.

1 bagel, any flavor (except cheese, egg, or chocolate chip!)
sliced fresh fruit (banana, orange, strawberries, peach, etc.)

Slice the bagel in half and toast it lightly. Place a layer (or several layers) of freshly sliced fruit on one half of the bagel and top it with the remaining half. Enjoy!

Per bagel: 265 calories; 7 g protein; 52 g carbohydrate; 1 g fat; 525 mg sodium; 0 mg cholesterol

Cinnamon Apple Oatmeal

Makes 3 cups

1 cup old fashioned rolled oats
1 green apple, cored and diced
¼ cup raisins
2 tablespoons chopped dates
¼ teaspoon cinnamon
¼ teaspoon salt
rice or soy milk for serving

Bring 2 cups of water to a boil, then add the oats, apple, raisins, dates, cinnamon, and salt. Bring to a simmer, then cook 3 minutes, stirring frequently. Remove from heat and cover. Allow to sit for 10 minutes. Spoon into bowls and serve with rice milk or soy milk.

Per 1 cup serving: 187 calories; 4 g protein; 38 g carbohydrate;
2 g fat; 181 mg sodium; 0 mg cholesterol

Quick Breakfast Rice

Makes about 4 cups

1½ cups vanilla soy milk
1 tablespoon cornstarch
2 cups cooked brown rice
¼ cup maple syrup
⅓ cup raisins
¼ teaspoon cinnamon
1 teaspoon vanilla

Pour vanilla soy milk into a medium-sized saucepan. Add the cornstarch and whisk until smooth. Stir in the rice, maple syrup, raisins and cinnamon. Bring to a simmer over medium heat.

Cook 3 minutes, then remove from heat and stir in the vanilla.

Serve hot or cold.

*Per 1 cup serving: 233 calories; 4 g protein; 51 g carbohydrate;
1 g fat; 170 mg sodium; 0 mg cholesterol*

Breakfast Cereals

Hot and cold cereals can provide a quick and wholesome breakfast if you choose your cereals carefully. When shopping for breakfast cereals, the old adage, "The simpler, the better," is helpful to keep in mind. Generally, the fewer ingredients in a breakfast cereal, the more healthful it will be.

When you read the ingredient list, the first ingredient should be a whole grain, or a mixture of whole grains, for example, whole wheat, corn, oats, barley, rice, etc. If the cereal includes salt, make sure it is only a small amount. Check the nutrition label. Ideally, a serving should contain 200 mg or less of sodium per serving.

Many cold cereals contain a lot of sugar, making them essentially a breakfast dessert. Check the ingredients. If sugar appears near the top of the list, or if there are several different forms of sugar included, such as dextrose, corn syrup, honey, barley malt, etc., then the cereal has too much sugar to be truly healthful. The major problem with these cereals is that you tend to eat more than you need, because it's difficult to stop eating sweets.

One other ingredient to watch for in cereals is fat, usually in the form of oil, or partially hydrogenated oil. One of the worst offenders in this category are the granola cereals, which often contain as much fat as many cookies. Cereals containing added fat should be avoided, because they will not help you lose weight. Instead, choose whole grain cereals with as little sugar as possible.

MUFFINS AND BREADS

Blueberry Muffins

Makes 12 muffins

1⅔ cups unbleached or whole wheat pastry flour
1½ teaspoons baking soda
½ teaspoon salt
½ teaspoon nutmeg
1 10.5-ounce package firm silken tofu
½ cup sugar
2 tablespoons orange juice concentrate
2 cups blueberries, fresh or frozen

Preheat oven to 350° F. Mix the flour, baking soda, salt, and nutmeg in a large bowl.

Place the tofu, sugar, and orange juice concentrate into a food processor and blend until completely smooth. Add to the flour mixture along with the blueberries and stir until just blended.

Drop spoonfuls of the batter into oil-sprayed muffin cups, and bake in the preheated oven for 25 minutes. Remove muffins from pan and cool on a rack.

Per muffin: 126 calories; 5 g protein; 25 g carbohydrate; 1 g fat; 195 mg sodium; 0 mg cholesterol

Banana Date Muffins

Makes 12 muffins

2 cups whole wheat pastry flour
2 teaspoons baking soda
½ teaspoon salt
⅓ cup wheat germ
⅓ cup oat bran
4 ripe bananas, mashed (about 2½ cups)
½ cup sugar
¾ cup soy milk or rice milk
1 teaspoon vanilla
⅓ cup chopped dates

Preheat oven to 350° F. Mix the flour, baking soda, salt, wheat germ, and oat bran in a large bowl.

In another bowl, mash the bananas and mix in the sugar. Stir in the soy milk and vanilla and mix thoroughly. Add the flour mixture, along with the dates, and stir to mix.

Fill oil-sprayed muffin cups nearly to the top, and bake in preheated oven for 20–30 minutes, until a toothpick inserted into the center comes out clean. Let stand 2 minutes, then remove muffins from pan and cool on a rack.

Per muffin: 174 calories; 5 g protein; 36 g carbohydrate; 1 g fat; 230 mg sodium; 0 mg cholesterol

Garlic Bread

Makes one loaf (about 20 slices)

Roasted garlic has a mellow flavor and creamy texture that makes delicious fat-free garlic bread.

2 large heads garlic
1 baguette or loaf of French bread, sliced
1-2 teaspoons mixed Italian herbs (optional)
¼ teaspoon salt

Roast the whole, unpeeled heads of garlic in a 400° F oven (or toaster oven) until they feel soft when squeezed. This will take about 30 minutes. Reduce the oven temperature to 350° F.

Peel the cloves or squeeze them out of their skin, then mash them into a paste with a fork. Mix in the herbs, if desired, and salt. Spread onto the sliced bread. Wrap tightly in foil and bake for 20 minutes.

Per slice: 91 calories; 3 g protein; 18.5 g carbohydrate; 0 g fat; 179 mg sodium; 0 mg cholesterol

Simple Bean Dip

Makes about 3 cups

1 15-ounce can fat-free refried beans
1-2 cups salsa (you choose the heat)
fresh cilantro
fat-free tortilla chips

Spoon the beans into a mixing bowl and stir in 1 cup of the salsa. Mix thoroughly. Transfer to a serving bowl and make a shallow depression in the top. Fill with salsa and garnish with fresh cilantro sprigs. Serve with fat-free tortilla chips.

Variation: For Simple Black Bean Dip, substitute one 15-ounce can of fat-free refried black beans in place of the refried beans.

Per tablespoon of dip: 23 calories; 1 g protein; 4 g carbohydrate; 0 g fat; 18 mg sodium; 0 mg cholesterol

Hummus

Makes about 2 cups

Hummus is a creamy garbanzo pâté that makes a delicious sandwich spread or dip with fresh vegetables or wedges of pita bread.

2 garlic cloves
1 tablespoon finely chopped parsley
1 15-ounce can garbanzo beans
1 tablespoon tahini (sesame seed butter)
2 tablespoons lemon juice
¼ teaspoon cumin
¼ teaspoon paprika
¼ teaspoon salt

Use a food processor to finely chop the garlic and parsley.

Drain the beans (save the liquid), and add them to the food processor along with the tahini, lemon juice, cumin, paprika, and salt. Process until very smooth. The mixture should be moist and spreadable. If it is too stiff, add some of the reserved bean liquid to achieve the desired consistency.

Per tablespoon: 27 calories; 1 g protein; 4 g carbohydrate; 0.5 g fat; 24 mg sodium; 0 mg cholesterol

SALAD DRESSINGS AND SALADS

Fat-free Salad Dressing

Makes ½ cup

Seasoned rice vinegar makes a simple, delicious dressing for salads and cooked vegetables. It will keep in the refrigerator for 2 to 3 weeks.

½ cup seasoned rice vinegar
1-2 teaspoons stone ground or Dijon mustard
1 garlic clove, pressed or crushed

Whisk all the ingredients together. Store in a closed jar or air-tight plastic container.

Per tablespoon: 14 calories; 0 g protein; 3 g carbohydrate; 0 g fat;
310 mg sodium; 0 mg cholesterol

Simple Piquant Dressing

Makes ½ cup

¼ cup of your favorite salsa
¼ cup seasoned rice vinegar

Mix the salsa and seasoned rice vinegar. Refrigerate any extra dressing.

Per 1 tablespoon: 8 calories; 0 g protein; 7 g carbohydrate;
0 g fat; 149 mg sodium; 0 mg cholesterol

Balsamic Vinaigrette

Makes ⅓ cup

Balsamic vinegar is a delicious wine vinegar from Italy with a mellow flavor that is perfect for salads.

2 tablespoons balsamic vinegar
2 tablespoons seasoned rice vinegar
2 tablespoons water
1-2 garlic cloves, crushed

Whisk all ingredients together.

Per 1 tablespoon: 6 calories; 0 g protein; 1.5 g carbohydrate; 0 g fat;
99 mg sodium; 0 mg cholesterol

Creamy Dill Dressing

Makes about 1½ cups

This rich-tasting, creamy dressing has no added oil. It is made with silken tofu which is available in most markets. Mori Nu is one popular brand.

    1 10.5-ounce package firm silken tofu
    1½ teaspoons garlic powder or granules
    ½ teaspoon dill weed
    ½ teaspoon salt
    2 tablespoons water
    1½ tablespoons lemon juice
    1 tablespoon seasoned rice vinegar

Combine all the ingredients in a food processor or blender and blend until completely smooth. Store any extra dressing in an airtight container in the refrigerator.

Per 1 tablespoon: 23 calories; 3 g protein; 2 g carbohydrate; 0.5 g fat; 115 mg sodium; 0 mg cholesterol

Cucumbers with Creamy Dill Dressing

Serves 6

1 batch Creamy Dill Dressing (preceding recipe)
2 cucumbers, peeled and thinly sliced
½ cup thinly sliced red onion

Combine all the ingredients in a salad bowl and toss to mix.

Per serving: 64 calories; 6 g protein; 7 g carbohydrate; 1 g fat;
232 mg sodium; 0 mg cholesterol

Mixed Greens Salad

Serves 6

For an almost instant salad, use one of the convenient prewashed salad mixes that are available in most markets. Add any other vegetables you enjoy (several are suggested below), and toss with fat-free dressing.

> 6 cups prewashed salad mix
> 1 tomato, cut into wedges
> ½ red or yellow bell pepper, seeded and sliced
> 1 carrot, grated or cut into thin slices
> ½ cup peeled and sliced jicama or cucumber
> 3 tablespoons fat-free dressing

Combine all ingredients and toss gently to mix.

Per serving: 20 calories; 0 g protein; 4 g carbohydrate; 0 g fat; 160 mg sodium; 0 mg cholesterol

South of the Border Salad

Serves 6

This salad is a cool and crunchy contrast to Mexican food or any other spicy cuisine. It may be made in advance and keeps well.

1 large carrot, peeled and cut into ¼-inch rounds
1 medium jicama, peeled and diced (about 2 cups)
1 red bell pepper, seeded and diced
1 small sweet onion, thinly sliced (about ½ cup)
2 tablespoons finely chopped cilantro
3 tablespoons Swanson's Vegetable Broth
2 tablespoons seasoned rice vinegar
2 tablespoons lemon juice
1 teaspoon stoneground mustard
¼ teaspoon salt
¼ teaspoon crushed red pepper flakes

Combine the carrot, jicama, bell pepper, onion, and cilantro in a salad bowl. In a small bowl, mix the remaining ingredients.

Pour over the vegetables and toss to mix.

Per serving: 32 calories; 1 g protein; 7 g carbohydrate; 0 g fat;
264 mg sodium; 0 mg cholesterol

Potato Salad

Serves 8

You'll love this delicious, old-fashioned potato salad without the added fat or cholesterol. Tofu is the secret for a creamy, nutritious dressing.

> **6 medium russet potatoes (about 8 cups diced)**
> **5 stalks celery, including leaves, thinly sliced**
> **1 small red onion, finely chopped**
> **1 cup finely chopped parsley**
> **1 cup finely shredded cabbage (optional)**
> **10.5-ounce package silken tofu**
> **⅓ cup seasoned rice vinegar**
> **¼ cup cider vinegar**
> **2 tablespoons stone ground mustard**
> **1 teaspoon dill weed**
> **1 teaspoon salt**
> **½ teaspoon black pepper**
> **½ teaspoon turmeric**

Scrub the potatoes, peel them if you wish, and cut them into cubes. Steam over boiling water until just tender, about 15 minutes, then transfer to a large bowl. Add the celery, onion, parsley, and cabbage.

In a blender, combine all the remaining ingredients. Blend until completely smooth, then pour over the salad. Toss gently to mix. Chill if time allows.

Per serving: 184 calories; 6 g protein; 38 g carbohydrate; 1 g fat; 461 mg sodium; 0 mg cholesterol

Tip: If the salad is kept for a while, the potatoes will absorb some of the dressing. You may wish to add a tablespoon or two of water to restore a moist, creamy texture.

Three Bean Salad

Serves 8

This salad is delicious all by itself or as an addition to a green salad.

> 1 15-ounce can kidney beans, drained
> 1 15-ounce can garbanzo beans, drained
> 1 15-ounce can green beans, drained
> ½ small red onion, finely chopped
> 4 tablespoons finely chopped fresh parsley
> ½ cup cider vinegar
> 2 tablespoons seasoned rice vinegar
> 3 garlic cloves, minced
> ½ teaspoon basil
> ¼ teaspoon each: oregano, marjoram, and black
> pepper

Drain the beans and toss them with the chopped onion and parsley.

In a separate bowl whisk the remaining ingredients together, then add to beans and toss to mix. Refrigerate and allow to marinate 2 to 3 hours before serving.

Per serving: 141 calories; 7 g protein; 26 g carbohydrate; 1 g fat;
140 mg of sodium; 0 mg cholesterol

Hoppin' John Salad

Makes about 6 cups

Black-eyed peas give this salad a wonderfully distinct flavor.

2 15-ounce cans black-eyed peas, drained
2 cups cooked brown rice
2 green onions, sliced
1-2 garlic cloves, crushed
1 stalk celery, sliced (about ½ cup)
2 small tomatoes, diced
2 tablespoons finely chopped parsley
⅓ cup lemon juice
½ teaspoon salt

Combine the black-eyed peas, cooked rice, green onions, garlic, celery, tomatoes, and chopped parsley in a salad bowl.

Mix the lemon juice and salt, then pour over the salad and toss gently to mix. Chill 1 to 2 hours if time permits.

Per serving: 110 calories; 5 g protein; 21 g carbohydrate; 0.5 g fat; 280 mg of sodium; 0 mg cholesterol

Ensalada de Frijoles

Serves 4

This recipe makes four very generous salads which are substantial enough to be a complete meal. The avocado adds wonderful flavor, a bit of fat, and vitamin E. Leave it out if you prefer.

2-3 cups cooked brown rice (page 132)
8 cups salad mix
2 carrots, grated or cut in thin strips
1 15-ounce can black beans, drained
1 cup diced jicama
2 tomatoes, sliced
1 15-ounce can corn, drained
½ cup cilantro leaves
½ avocado, thinly sliced (optional)
¼ cup of your favorite salsa
¼ cup seasoned rice vinegar
1 garlic clove, crushed or pressed
additional salsa for topping

Heat the brown rice and make a bed of it on each of four plates. Top with a layer of salad mix and grated carrot. Rinse the beans, then sprinkle them over each of the salads. Add the jicama, tomatoes, corn, cilantro, and avocado. Mix the salsa, seasoned rice vinegar, and crushed garlic. Sprinkle over the salad, then top with a generous spoonful of salsa.

Per serving (with avocado): 344 calories; 11 g protein;
63 g carbohydrate; 5 g fat; 357 mg sodium; 0 mg cholesterol

Per serving (without avocado): 302 calories; 10 g protein;
60 g carbohydrate; 2 g fat; 355 mg sodium; 0 mg cholesterol

Soups

Tomato Soup

Serves 6 to 8

Hot, steamy tomato soup is one of everyone's favorite foods. This quick version is made with canned tomatoes and takes just 20 minute to prepare.

1 small onion, chopped
3 stalks celery, sliced
1 28-ounce can crushed tomatoes, including liquid
2½ teaspoons sugar
½ teaspoon paprika
½ teaspoon basil
¼ teaspoon pepper
3 cups soy milk
1 cup cooked brown rice
½ teaspoon salt

Combine the onion, celery, tomatoes, sugar, paprika, basil, and pepper in a pot. Cover and simmer 15 minutes, stirring occasionally. Transfer 3 cups of the soup to a blender. Add the soymilk and blend until smooth. Return to the pot and add the rice and salt. Heat over a low flame until very hot and steamy.

Per serving: 137 calories; 4 g protein; 28 g carbohydrate; 1 g fat; 265 mg sodium; 0 mg cholesterol

Potato and Corn Chowder

Serves 8

This is a mildly spicy chowder that is delicious with cornbread and a green salad with Simple Piquant Dressing (page 115).

4 russet potatoes, peeled and diced (about 4 cups)
2½ cups water or vegetable stock
1 yellow onion, chopped
2 garlic cloves, minced
1 red bell pepper, diced
1 teaspoon ground cumin
1 teaspoon basil
1 teaspoon salt
¼ teaspoon black pepper
1 4-ounce can diced chilies
2 cups corn, fresh or frozen
1-2 cups soy milk

Combine the diced potatoes in a pot with 2 cups of water or vegetable stock. Cover and cook until tender, about 20 minutes.

Heat the remaining ½ cup of water or stock in a large pot and cook the onion, garlic, and bell pepper for 3 minutes. Add the cumin, basil, salt, and pepper and continue to cook until the onion is very soft, about 5 more minutes.

When the potatoes are tender, mash them in their water, and combine them with the onion mixture, along with the diced chilies, corn and 1 cup of the soy milk. Stir to blend. Add more soy milk if the soup is too thick. Heat gently until hot and steamy.

For a milder soup, use only half of the chilies. Freeze the rest for later use.

Per serving: 179 calories; 4 g protein; 40 g carbohydrate; 0.5 g fat;
305 mg sodium; 0 mg cholesterol

Golden Mushroom Soup

Serves 6

This is a rich-tasting soup, delicious with fresh baked bread, baked yams, and a green salad.

> 2½ cups water or vegetable stock
> 2 tablespoons soy sauce
> 2 medium onions, chopped
> 1 pound mushrooms, sliced
> 1½ teaspoons dill weed
> 1 tablespoon paprika
> 1 teaspoon caraway seeds (optional)
> ⅛ teaspoon pepper
> 1½ cups soy milk
> 2 teaspoons lemon juice
> 2-3 tablespoons red wine (optional)

Heat ½ cup of the water or vegetable stock in a large pot. Add 1 tablespoon of the soy sauce along with the chopped onions and cook until the onions are soft and translucent, about 5 minutes.

Add the sliced mushrooms, dill, paprika, caraway seeds, an pepper, and cook another 5 minutes, stirring frequently. Add remaining water or stock and soy sauce, then cover and simmer for 15 minutes.

Place 1 cup of the soup into a blender, along with the soy milk, and blend until smooth. Return it to the pot and heat, without boiling, until steamy. Stir in the lemon juice and red wine just before serving.

Per serving: 81 calories; 3 g protein; 14 g carbohydrate; 0.5 g fat; 229 mg sodium; 0 mg cholesterol

Minestrone

Serves 8

This tomato-vegetable soup is delicious as is, or enhance it with additional vegetables of your choosing. Add fresh-baked bread or muffins and a salad for a satisfying meal.

> 1 small onion, chopped
> 2 garlic cloves, minced
> 1 carrot, cut into chunks
> 2 stalks celery, sliced including tops
> 2 cup finely shredded green cabbage
> 2 medium potatoes, scrubbed and cut into chunks
> 2 tablespoons chopped parsley
> 4 cups tomato juice
> 4 cups water or vegetable stock
> 2 teaspoons dried basil
> 2 teaspoons mixed Italian herbs
> ⅛ teaspoon cayenne
> 1 medium zucchini, diced
> ½ cup pasta shells
> 1 15-ounce can cannelini beans, drained
> 1-2 cups finely chopped kale, collard greens, or
>   spinach.

Chop the onion, garlic, carrot, celery, cabbage, potatoes, an parsley. Place in a large pot with the tomato juice, water or stock, basil, Italian herbs, and cayenne. Bring to a simmer, then cover and cook 20 minutes.

Add the zucchini, pasta, cannelini beans, and chopped greens, then cover and simmer an additional 20 minutes, until the pasta is tender. Add extra tomato juice or water if the soup becomes too thick.

Per serving: 158 calories; 6 g protein; 33 g carbohydrate; 0 g fat; 347 mg sodium; 0 mg cholesterol

Borscht

Serves 8

2 beets, peeled and diced
1 medium onion chopped
2 medium potatoes, cut in ½-inch cubes
2 carrots, sliced or diced
3 celery stalks, sliced
2 cups finely shredded green cabbage
2 15-ounce cans Swanson's Vegetable Broth
1 15-ounce can crushed tomatoes
4 cups water
1 teaspoon dill weed
½ teaspoon caraway seeds
¼ teaspoon black pepper
1 cup sauerkraut

Combine everything except the sauerkraut in a large pot and bring to a simmer. Cover and cook until the beets and potatoes are tender, about 20 minutes.

Stir in the sauerkraut and serve.

Per serving: 97 calories; 2 g protein; 22 g carbohydrate; 0 g fat; 366 mg sodium; 0 mg cholesterol

Green Velvet Soup

Serves 10

This beautiful green soup is a delicious way to eat your vegetables.

1 onion, chopped
2 stalks celery, sliced
2 potatoes, scrubbed and diced
¾ cup split peas, rinsed
2 bay leaves
6 cups water or vegetable stock
2 medium zucchini, diced
1 medium stalk broccoli, chopped
1 bunch fresh spinach, washed and chopped
½ teaspoon basil
¼ teaspoon black pepper
1 teaspoon salt

Place onion, celery, potatoes, split peas and bay leaves in a large pot with water or stock and bring to a boil. Lower heat, cover, and simmer 1 hour. Remove bay leaves. Add zucchini, broccoli, spinach, basil, and black pepper, and simmer 20 minutes. Transfer to a blender in several small batches and blend until completely smooth, holding the lid on tightly.

Return to pot and heat until steamy. Add salt to taste.

Per serving: 120 calories; 5 g protein; 24 g carbohydrate; 0 g fat; 238 mg sodium; 0 mg cholesterol

Curried Sweet Potato Soup

Serves 8

Yams take on a whole different character in this spicy, slightly sweet soup.

> **2 medium yams**
> **½ cup water**
> **1 onion chopped**
> **½ teaspoon each: mustard seeds, turmeric, ginger, and cumin**
> **¼ teaspoon cinnamon**
> **⅛ teaspoon cayenne**
> **¾ teaspoon salt**
> **2 cups water**
> **1 tablespoon lemon juice**
> **2 cups soy milk**

Peel the yams and cut them into chunks. Steam over boiling water until tender when pierced with a fork, about 40 minutes. Mash (you should have about 2 cups), and set aside.

Braise the onion in ½ cup water until soft, then add the spices and salt. Cook 2 minutes over low heat, stirring constantly, then whisk in 2 cups water, lemon juice, and mashed yams. Simmer 10 minutes. Add soy milk and puree soup in a blender in two to three batches until very smooth. Return to the pan and heat over a medium flame until hot and steamy, about 10 minutes.

Per serving: 82 calories; 2 g protein; 18 g carbohydrate; 0.5 g fat; 227 mg of sodium; 0 mg cholesterol

Okefenokee Stew

Serves 8

This delicious, easy-to-prepare stew was inspired by a balmy southern evening in the Okefenokee Swamp. For traditional southern flavors, what better than okra and black eye peas?

½ cup red wine
1 large onion, chopped
1 bell pepper, diced
2 stalks celery, sliced
3-4 cups sliced okra (¾ to 1 pound)
1 15-ounce can chopped tomatoes
2 teaspoons each: chili powder and oregano
1 tablespoon soy sauce
1 can black eye peas, with liquid
2 cups frozen corn

Heat wine in a large pot and cook chopped onion until tender, about 5 minutes. Add celery, bell pepper, okra, tomatoes and seasonings. Lower heat, cover and simmer 10 minutes. Add black eye peas and corn and simmer 5 to 10 minutes longer. Serve over cooked brown rice.

Per serving: 126 calories; 5 g protein; 24 g carbohydrate; 0 g fat; 324 mg of sodium; 0 mg cholesterol

GRAINS

Brown Rice

Makes 3 cups of cooked rice

Whole grains are the foundation of a healthful diet, and brown rice is a great grain to start with. It has a crunchy, nut-like flavor and supplies more vitamins, minerals, protein, and fiber than white rice. Cooking it in extra water guarantees perfect rice every time.

> **1 cup short grain brown rice**
> **4 cups water**
> **½ teaspoon salt**

Rinse and drain rice. In a saucepan bring the water to a boil, then add the rice and salt. When the water begins to boil again, lower the heat slightly, then cover and simmer about 40 minutes, until the rice is soft but still retains a hint of crunchiness.

Pour off any excess liquid (this can be saved and used as a broth for soups and stews if desired).

Per ½ cup: 115 calories; 2 g protein; 25 g carbohydrate; 0.5 g fat; 176 mg sodium; 0 mg cholesterol

Wild Basmati Pilaf

Serves 6

Wild rice and basmati rice add wonderful flavor and texture to this fat-free pilaf. Look for both in natural food stores and in some supermarkets. Serve this pilaf with everyday meals or as an elegant sidedish.

¼ cup wild rice
1 15-ounce can Swanson's Vegetable Broth
¾ cups brown basmati rice
1 onion, finely chopped
3 garlic cloves, minced
2 cups thinly sliced mushrooms
2 stalks celery, thinly sliced
½ teaspoon thyme
½ teaspoon marjoram
¼ teaspoon black pepper
¼ teaspoon salt
⅓ cup finely chopped parsley

Rinse the wild rice and place it in a saucepan with the vegetable broth and ½ cup of water. Stir to mix, then cover and simmer for 20 minutes. At the end of this time, add the basmati rice.

Cover and continue cooking until both varieties of rice are tender, about 50 minutes.

Heat ½ cup of water in a large pot or skillet. Add the onion and garlic and cook until all the water has evaporated and browned bits of onion begin to stick to the pan. Add another ¼ cup of water, scrape the pan, and cook until the onions begin to stick again. Repeat this process of adding water and cooking the onions until they are nicely browned. This will take about 15 minutes.

Stir in the mushrooms, celery, and seasonings. Cook, stirring frequently, for 5 minutes, then add the cooked rice and finely chopped parsley. Cook over low heat, turning gently, until the mixture is very hot.

Per serving: 124 calories; 3 g protein; 27 g carbohydrate; 0.5 g fat;
284 mg sodium; 0 mg cholesterol

Simple Spanish Rice

Makes 2½ cups

Here is a simple Spanish rice recipe that's baked in the oven. Spike is a seasoning salt available in most markets in the spice section.

1 cup brown basmati rice (or other long grain brown rice)
2¼ cups boiling water or vegetable stock
2½ tablespoons soy sauce
1 teaspoon chili powder
½ teaspoon Spike seasoning or ¼ teaspoon salt
¼ teaspoon cumin
¼ teaspoon garlic powder

Preheat the oven to 350° F. Spread the rice in a 9 x 9-inch baking dish. Combine the boiling water or stock with the remaining ingredients and pour over the rice. Cover tightly with foil and bake in preheated oven until the rice is tender and all the water is absorbed, about 1 hour.

Per ½ cup: 105 calories; 3 g protein; 23 g carbohydrate; 0 g fat; 341 mg sodium; 0 mg cholesterol

Bulgur

Makes about 3 cups

Bulgur is cracked wheat which has been toasted to give it a delicious, nutty flavor. It cooks in about 15 minutes and is an excellent accompaniment to a wide variety of foods, from chili to roasted vegetables. If you like, season it with chili powder, curry powder, or soy sauce. Or you can add it to soups, stews, and chili for extra flavor and texture, serve it as a hot breakfast cereal, or mix it with chopped fresh vegetables and fat-free dressing for a delicious salad.

2 cups water
1 cup bulgur
½ teaspoon salt

Bring water to a boil in a saucepan, then stir in bulgur and salt. Reduce heat to a simmer, then cover and cook until bulgur is tender, about 15 minutes.

Per ½ cup: 113 calories; 4 g protein; 24 g carbohydrate; 0 g fat; 181 mg sodium; 0 mg cholesterol

Alternate method: Stir bulgur and salt together in a mixing bowl. Stir in boiling water. Cover and let stand until the liquid is absorbed and the bulgur is tender, about 20 minutes.

Couscous

Makes 3 cups

Couscous, which is actually a type of pasta, cooks in minutes and makes a delicious side dish or salad. Many natural food stores sell whole wheat couscous, which has a nuttier flavor and more fiber than regular couscous. They are both prepared in the manner described below.

1½ cups boiling water
½ teaspoon salt
1 cup couscous (whole wheat or regular)

Bring salted water to a boil in a small pan. Stir in the couscous, then remove the pan from heat and cover it. Let stand 10 to 15 minutes, then fluff with a fork and serve.

Per ½ cup: 91 calories; 3 g protein; 20 g carbohydrate; 0 g fat; 181 mg sodium; 0 mg cholesterol

Polenta

Makes 2 cups

Polenta, or coarsely ground cornmeal, has long been a staple grain in northern Italy. It cooks easily and is delicious with marinara or any other spicy sauce. Pour the cooked polenta onto a platter and top it with sauce, or spoon it into a flat dish and chill it, then slice and grill it as described below.

½ cup polenta
1 15-ounce can Swanson's Vegetable Broth
½ cup water

Combine the polenta, vegetable broth, and ½ cup of water in a saucepan. Bring to a simmer and cook, stirring frequently, until very thick, 15 to 20 minutes. Pour into a 9 x 9-inch baking dish and chill completely. Cut into squares and grill or saute in an oil-sprayed nonstick skillet.

Per ½ cup: 62 calories; 1 g protein; 14 g carbohydrate; 0 g fat; 437 mg sodium; 0 mg cholesterol

Quinoa

Makes 3 cups

Quinoa, pronounced "keen-wah," is a light fluffy grain which makes a delicious breakfast cereal, side dish, or salad. It cooks in just fifteen minutes and is a rich source of many nutrients, including protein, B vitamins, and iron. Look for quinoa in your favorite natural food store.

1 cup quinoa
2 cups water

Rinse the quinoa thoroughly by placing it in a bowl and adding about 3 cups of cold water. Swish it around until the water is cloudy, then pour it into a strainer. Put it back into the bowl and rinse it again. Repeat the process 3 or 4 times until the water remains clear.

Place the rinsed quinoa into a pan and add 2 cups of cold water.

Bring to a boil, then reduce the heat to a simmer. Cover and cook until all the water is absorbed, about 15 minutes

*Per ½ cup: 118 calories; 5 g protein; 20 g carbohydrate; 2 g fat;
3 mg sodium; 0 mg cholesterol*

Favorite Bread Stuffing

Serves 8

You'll love this traditional stuffing now that it's fat-free!

½ cup water
1 onion, chopped
3 cups sliced mushrooms (about ½ pound)
2 celery stalks, thinly sliced
4 cups cubed bread
⅓ cup finely chopped parsley
½ teaspoon thyme
½ teaspoon marjoram
½ teaspoon sage
⅛ teaspoon black pepper
½ teaspoon salt
1 cup very hot water or vegetable stock

Heat ½ cup water in a large pot or skillet. Add the onion and cook 5 minutes.

Add the sliced mushrooms and celery and cook over medium heat, stirring occasionally, until the mushrooms begin to brown, about 5 minutes.

Preheat the oven to 350° F. Stir in the bread, parsley, thyme, marjoram, sage, black pepper, and salt. Lower the heat and continue cooking for 3 minutes, then stir in the water or stock, a little at a time, until the dressing obtains the desired moistness. Spread in an oil-sprayed baking dish, cover and bake for 20 minutes. Remove the cover and bake 10 minutes longer.

Per serving: 91 calories; 3 g protein; 14 g carbohydrate; 2 g fat;
297 mg sodium; 0 mg cholesterol

VEGETABLE DISHES

Braised Cabbage

Serves 4

Adrien Avis provided this simple and delicious vegetable dish.

½ cup water
2 cups cabbage, coarsely chopped
½ teaspoon caraway seeds (optional)
salt and fresh ground black pepper

Bring the water to a boil in a skillet or saucepan and add the cabbage and caraway seeds. Cover and cook until just tender, about 5 minutes. Sprinkle with salt and black pepper and serve.

Per serving: 16 calories; 0.5 g protein; 4 g carbohydrate; 0 g fat; 13 mg sodium; 0 mg cholesterol

Steamed Kale

Serves 2 to 4

If you've never tried kale, you're in for a treat. Besides being delicious, kale is an excellent source of calcium and beta carotene. This is the simplest method I know of preparing it.

1 bunch of kale (6 to 8 cups chopped)
½ cup water
2 teaspoons soy sauce
2-3 garlic cloves, minced

Wash the kale, remove the stems, and chop the leaves into ½-inch wide strips.

Heat the water and soy sauce in a large pot or skillet. Add the garlic and cook it 1 to 2 minutes. Add the chopped kale and toss to mix. Cover and cook over medium heat until tender, about 5 minutes.

Per 1 cup: 61 calories; 3 g protein; 11 g carbohydrate; 0 g fat;
101 mg sodium; 0 mg cholesterol

Potatoes with Kale and Corn

Serves 6

4 russet potatoes
1 bunch kale
½ cup water
2-3 teaspoons soy sauce
3 garlic cloves, minced
1 15-ounce can corn, including liquid

Scrub the potatoes, cut them into cubes, and steam them over boiling water until tender, about 15 minutes.

Wash the kale and remove the stems. Chop the leaves into small pieces. Heat ½ cup of water and 2 teaspoons of soy sauce in a large pan, then add the garlic. Cook 1 minute, then add the chopped kale. Toss to mix, then cover and cook over medium heat until the kale is tender, about 5 minutes. Add the corn with its liquid, and the cooked potatoes. Stir to mix.

Per serving: 238 calories; 5 g protein; 52 g carbohydrate; 0.5 g fat;
120 mg sodium; 0 mg cholesterol

Mashed Potatoes and Gravy

Serves 8

This is a simple, fat-free version of a traditional favorite.

4 large russet potatoes, peeled and diced
2 cups water
½ teaspoon salt
½-1 cup soy milk or rice milk
½ cup water
1 tablespoon soy sauce
½ cup finely chopped onion
1 cup sliced mushrooms
2 tablespoons flour
½ cup water
¼ teaspoon garlic powder or granules
¼ teaspoon poultry seasoning
⅛ teaspoon black pepper

Simmer the potatoes in 2 cups of salted water until tender, about 10 minutes. Drain and reserve the liquid. Mash the potatoes, adding enough milk to achieve desired consistency. Add salt to taste. Cover and set aside.

Heat ½ cup of water and soy sauce in a large skillet, then add onions and mushrooms. Cover and cook over medium heat 5 minutes, stirring occasionally.

Mix the flour with ½ cup water and add it to the onions along with the seasonings and reserved potato water. Stir over medium heat until thickened.

Per serving: 134 calories; 3 g protein; 30 g carbohydrate; 0 g fat; 228 mg sodium; 0 mg cholesterol

Baked Yams

Serves 4

Yams are a great year-round food. Delicious and easy to prepare, they are loaded with beneficial nutrients like beta-carotene, potassium, and fiber. Serve them with meals and keep them on hand for snacks. Eat them plain, or topped with a bit of maple syrup or applesauce.

4 medium yams (jewel and garnet yams are especially flavorful)

Microwave oven: Scrub the yams but do not peel them. Prick them in several places with a fork or sharp knife. Place two yams in the microwave and cook on high for 6 minutes. Turn the yams over and cook an additional 6 minutes. The yams are done when they are easily pierced with a fork.

Conventional oven: Scrub and prick the yams as above. Line the bottom of a baking dish with foil or baking parchment, then place the yams in the dish and bake at 400° F for 1 hour, or until tender when pierced with a fork.

Per yam: 158 calories; 1.5 g protein; 38 g carbohydrate; 0 g fat;
12 mg sodium; 0 mg cholesterol

Lasagne

Serves 10

½ cup water or red wine
1 onion, chopped
1 carrot, grated
3 garlic cloves, minced
2 cups mushrooms, sliced
1 15-oz. can tomatoes, chopped with their juice
1 28-oz. can tomato sauce
1 teaspoon each: basil, oregano
½ teaspoon each: thyme, fennel seed
⅛ teaspoon cayenne
1 lb. firm tofu, mashed
½ cup chopped fresh parsley
2 tablespoon soy sauce
1 10-ounce package frozen chopped spinach,
   thawed
12 ounces lasagne noodles (about 10 noodles),
   uncooked

Saute the onion and carrot in ½ cup water or red wine until soft, about 5 minutes, then add the garlic and mushrooms. Continue cooking until mushrooms are brown, about 5 minutes. Stir in the tomatoes, tomato sauce, and seasonings and simmer 20 minutes. While the sauce simmers, combine the mashed tofu, chop-ped parsley, and soy sauce.

To assemble the lasagne, spread about ½ cup of the sauce over the bottom of a 9 x 12-inch baking dish. Cover with a layer of uncooked noodles, then with ½ of the tofu mixture and half of the spinach. Spread ½ of the remaining sauce over this. Now make layers with the remaining noodles, tofu mixture, spinach, and sauce. Cover tightly with foil, and bake at 350x for 1 hour, or until the noodles are tender.

Let stand 10 minutes before serving.

Per serving: 176 calories; 12 g protein; 27 g carbohydrate; 2 g fat; 253 mg sodium; 0 mg cholesterol

HEARTIER DISHES

Super Spaghetti

Serves 8

Spaghetti doesn't get any easier, unless you buy it ready-made! This simple, tasty sauce goes well with manicotti, lasagne, or any other pasta dish.

> 8 ounces spaghetti
> ½ cup red or white wine or water
> 1 onion, chopped
> 4 garlic cloves, crushed
> 2 cups sliced mushrooms
> 1 28-ounce can crushed tomatoes
> 1 tablespoon mixed Italian Herbs
> 1 teaspoon sugar
> ½ teaspoon fennel seeds (optional)
> ¼ teaspoon black pepper

Cook the spaghetti until it is tender. Drain and rinse. Set aside.

While the spaghetti cooks, heat the wine or water in a large pot, add the onion, garlic, and mushrooms. Cook until the onion is soft and translucent, about 5 minutes. Add the remaining ingredients and simmer for 15 to 20 minutes.

Spread the cooked spaghetti on a platter and top with the sauce.

Per ½ cup: 103 calories; 4 g protein; 18 g carbohydrate; 0 g fat; 255 mg sodium; 0 mg cholesterol

Polenta
with Hearty Barbecue Sauce

Serves 8

Textured vegetable protein (TVP) provides a meaty flavor with none of meat's fat or cholesterol. You'll find it in natural food stores.

> 3 teaspoons soy sauce
> 1 large onion, finely chopped
> 1 bell pepper, finely diced
> 3 large garlic cloves, minced
> 1 15-ounce can tomato sauce
> 1 cup textured vegetable protein (TVP)
> 1 tablespoon sugar
> 1 teaspoon chili powder
> 2 tablespoons cider vinegar
> 1 tablespoon peanut butter
> 1 teaspoon stone ground or Dijon-style mustard
> 4 cups cooked polenta (1 cup uncooked) (page 138)

Heat ½ cup of water and 1 teaspoon of soy sauce in a large pot.

Add the onion, bell pepper, and garlic and cook until the onion is soft, about 5 minutes. Add the tomato sauce, TVP, sugar, chili powder, vinegar, peanut butter, mustard, and 1 cup of water. Cook over medium heat, stirring frequently, until the TVP is softened and the sauce is thick, about 10 minutes.

Spread the cooked polenta onto a serving bowl or platter, then top with sauce and serve.

Per serving: 146 calories; 8 g protein; 24 g carbohydrate; 1 g fat; 215 mg of sodium; 0 mg cholesterol

Sweet and Sour Vegetable Stir-Fry

Serves 4

⅓ cup ketchup
⅓ cup vinegar
⅓ cup brown sugar
1 tablespoon soy sauce
1 tablespoon cornstarch
¼ teaspoon dried red pepper flakes
½ cup water
½ cup water or vegetable stock
1 cup thinly sliced onion
2 garlic cloves, crushed
2 cups sliced mushrooms
1 red bell pepper, thinly sliced
1 medium zucchini, thinly sliced
2 cups snow peas
3-4 cups cooked rice (page 132)

Combine the ketchup, vinegar, brown sugar, soy sauce, cornstarch, pepper flakes, and ½ cup of water in a small bowl. Stir to mix, then set aside. In a large skillet or wok, heat ½ cup of water or vegetable stock and add the onion and garlic. Cook until the onion begins to soften, about 3 minutes. Add the mushrooms and cook 3 minutes, then add the bell pepper and zucchini. Continue cooking over medium-high heat, stirring continuously, until the vegetables are just becoming tender, about 3 minutes. Add the snowpeas and reserved sauce mixture and cook, stirring constantly, until the sauce is clear and thickened, about 2 minutes.

Serve over cooked rice.

Per serving: 352 calories; 8 g protein; 73 g carbohydrate; 3 g fat; 320 mg sodium; 0 mg cholesterol

Fast Lane Chow Mein

Serves 4 to 6

This chow mein takes just minutes to prepare and is a delicious way to load up on nutritious vegetables.

½ cup water
2 teaspoons soy sauce
1 onion, chopped
4-5 garlic cloves, minced
1 cup thinly sliced green cabbage
1 stalk celery, thinly sliced
1 pound sliced mushrooms, fresh or frozen
3 cups chopped kale
2 packages vegetarian ramen soup (I use
    Westbrae Miso Ramen)
1 cup water

Heat ½ cup of water and 1 teaspoon of soy sauce in a large pot. Add the chopped onion and garlic. Cook until the onion is soft, about 5 minutes. Add the cabbage, celery, mushrooms, and kale.

Crush the ramen noodles (I use the handle of my knife to do this) and add them to the vegetable mixture along with one of the ramen seasoning packets and 1 cup of water. Stir to mix, then cover and cook over medium heat, stirring occasionally, until the vegetables and noodles are tender, about 5 minutes. Check the seasonings and add a bit more of the ramen seasoning mix if needed.

Per serving: 163 calories; 6 g protein; 32 g carbohydrate; 1 g fat;
*   594 mg sodium; 0 mg cholesterol*

Thai Vegetables with Rice

Serves 8

In this dish, colorful vegetables are simmered in a flavorful sauce and served over aromatic basmati or jasmine rice. For a mild dish, use the smaller amount of dried red pepper flakes. Increase the amount for a more fiery version.

½ cup water
2 tablespoons soy sauce
1 onion, thinly sliced
4 garlic cloves, minced
1 pound yams, peeled and cut into wedges
1 15-ounce can crushed tomatoes
2 teaspoons ground coriander
1 teaspoon ground cumin
½-1 teaspoon red pepper flakes
½ teaspoon turmeric
½ teaspoon ginger powder (or 2 teaspoons fresh
    ginger, grated)
½ cup water

1 15-ounce can garbanzo beans, including liquid
½ pound fresh green beans, trimmed and cut into
    1-inch pieces (about 2 cups)
1 red bell pepper, cut into thin strips
2 teaspoons grated lemon rind (lemon zest)
1 tablespoon lemon juice
1 tablespoon soy sauce
6 cups cooked basmati or jasmine rice (2 cups raw)

Heat ½ cup of water and 1 tablespoon of soy sauce in a large pot. Add the chopped onion and garlic. Cook until the onion is very soft, about 5 minutes. Add the yam, crushed tomatoes, coriander, cumin, red pepper flakes, turmeric, ginger, and ½ cup of water. Cover and simmer 5 minutes.

Add the garbanzo beans with their liquid and the green beans, then cover and simmer 5 more minutes. Add the bell pepper and lemon rind and simmer until the yams and green beans are tender when pierced with a sharp knife, about 10 minutes. Stir in the lemon juice and remaining soy sauce. Serve over cooked rice.

Per serving: 286 calories; 7 g protein; 62 g carbohydrate; 1 g fat; 166 mg sodium; 0 mg cholesterol

Chili Mac

Serves 8

Kids love this easy-to-make meal.

8 ounces pasta spirals
½ cup water
1 onion, chopped
1 small bell pepper, diced
3 garlic cloves, minced
¾ cup textured vegetable protein
1 28-ounce can crushed tomatoes
1 15-ounce can kidney beans, including liquid
1 15-ounce can corn, including liquid
¾ cup water
2 teaspoons ground cumin
4-6 teaspoons chili powder
½ teaspoon salt

Cook the pasta in boiling water until it is tender. Drain and rinse it, then set it aside.

Heat ½ cup of water in a large pot then add the onion, bell pepper, and garlic. Cook until the onion is soft, about 5 minutes. Add the textured vegetable protein, crushed tomatoes, kidney beans, corn, and an additional ¾ cup of water. Stir in the cumin, chili powder, and salt, then simmer over medium heat, stirring occasionally, for 20 minutes. Stir in the cooked pasta and check the seasonings. Add more chili powder if a spicier dish is desired.

Per serving: 170 calories; 9 g protein; 32 g carbohydrate; 1 g fat;
434 mg sodium; 0 mg cholesterol

Fat-Free Hot Dogs and Burgers

Now you and your family can enjoy delicious vegetarian hot dogs, chili dogs, and burgers without any fat or cholesterol. Look for Smart Dogs, Yve's Veggie Wieners, or Garden Dogs in your supermarket or natural food store. Delicious vegetarian burger patties are available in many supermarkets and natural food stores.

Brands vary in flavor and texture, so do some exploring to find your favorites. Some of my favorites are the Garden Vegan by Wholesome and Hearty Foods, the Boca Burger by the Boca Burger Company, and the Natural Touch Burger by Morningstar Farms. Be sure to select varieties that are low in fat (3 grams or less per patty). You may also want to try using vegetarian burgers in place of meat in sauces, stuffings, and tacos (see the recipe for Tacos on page 157).

Chili Burger Deluxe

Makes enough for 2 burgers

Use one of the delicious fat-free, meatless patties listed above for this great-tasting burger.

> **2 vegetarian burger patties**
> **1 burger bun, preferably whole grain**
> **1 15-ounce can vegetarian chili beans**
> **2 tomato slices**
> **barbecue sauce or salsa**

For each burger you are making, heat one patty in a toaster oven, microwave, or in a skillet, lightly toast one half of a burger bun, and heat about 1 cup of chili beans on the stove or in a microwave.

To assemble, top the bun half with a burger patty, a tomato slice, and the heated chili beans. Garnish with barbecue sauce or salsa.

Per burger: 352 calories; 24 g protein; 60 g carbohydrate; 1 g fat; 566 mg sodium; 0 mg cholesterol

Tacos

Makes 12 tacos

Boca Burgers are fat-free, meatless patties, available in natural food stores and in a growing number of supermarkets. If you are unable to locate Boca Burgers, substitute any other fat-free vegetarian burger.

½ cup water
½ onion, chopped
3 garlic cloves, crushed
1 small bell pepper, finely diced
½ cup tomato sauce
4 Boca Burgers, thawed and crumbled
2 teaspoons chili powder
½ teaspoon cumin
½ teaspoon oregano

12 corn tortillas
1 cup shredded leaf lettuce
1 medium tomato, diced
4 green onions, sliced
½ cup salsa or taco sauce

Heat ½ cup of water in a large skillet and cook onion, garlic and pepper until the onion is soft, about 5 minutes. Stir in the tomato sauce, crumbled Boca Burgers, chili powder, cumin, and oregano. Cook over low heat until the mixture is fairly dry, about 3 minutes.

To assemble the tacos, place a small amount of filling on a tortilla and place it in a heavy, ungreased skillet. Heat until the tortilla is soft and warm, then fold in half and cook on each side for 60 seconds or longer for a crisper taco. Garnish with remaining ingredients.

Per taco: 114 calories; 7 g protein; 19 g carbohydrate; 1 g fat;
86 mg sodium; 0 mg cholesterol

Broccoli Burritos

Makes 6 burritos

This delicious dish turns broccoli into a meal. Roasted red peppers are available in jars in most markets, and tahini is sold in natural food stores, ethnic markets, and many supermarkets.

1 bunch of broccoli
1 15-ounce can garbanzo beans
½ cup roasted red peppers
2 tablespoons tahini (sesame seed butter)
3 tablespoons lemon juice
6 flour tortillas
6 tablespoons salsa (more or less to taste)

Cut or break the broccoli into flowerets. Peel the stalks and cut them into ½-inch thick rounds. You should have about 2 cups. Steam over boiling water until just tender, about 5 minutes.

Drain the garbanzo beans and place them in a food processor with the peppers, tahini, and lemon juice. Process until very smooth.

Spread about ¼ cup of the garbanzo mixture on a tortilla and place it face up in a large heated skillet. Heat it until the tortilla is warm and soft, about 2 minutes. Spread a line of broccoli down the center of the tortilla and sprinkle with salsa.

Fold the bottom of the tortilla up, then starting on one side, roll the tortilla around the broccoli. Repeat with the remaining tortillas.

Per burrito: 244 calories; 9 g protein; 39 g carbohydrate; 5 g fat; 130 mg sodium; 0 mg cholesterol

Tip: You can reduce the fat content by using fat-free flour tortillas which are sold in many supermarkets. Or try using chapatis (Indian flatbreads), which are made with whole wheat flour and are usually fat-free. Look for them in your favorite natural food store.

Quick Black Bean Chili

Serves 6

There are so many ways to enjoy delicious Black Bean Chili: serve it with brown rice and a green salad, use it as a filling for burritos, or try it over potatoes, as suggested in the next recipe. For a hotter chili, add some cayenne or fresh chopped jalapenos.

½ cup water
1 tablespoon soy sauce
2 onions, chopped
4 garlic cloves, crushed
2 15-ounce cans black beans
1 15-ounce can crushed tomatoes
1 4-ounce can diced chilies
2 teaspoons oregano
½ teaspoon cumin
¼ teaspoon salt
fresh cilantro, chopped

Heat the water and soy sauce in a large pan, then add the onion and garlic and cook until the onion is soft, about 5 minutes.

Add the black beans with their liquid, the tomatoes, chilies, oregano, cumin, and salt. Cover and simmer 25 minutes. Top with chopped fresh cilantro and serve.

Per serving: 138 calories; 7 g protein; 26 g carbohydrate; 0 g fat;
199 mg sodium; 0 mg cholesterol

Potatoes with Black Bean Chili

Makes 4 potatoes

4 red or yellow potatoes
1 cup black bean chili, homemade or commercial
½ cup salsa
2 green onions, sliced
¼ cup chopped cilantro

Scrub the potatoes and steam them until they are just tender when pierced with a fork, about 35 minutes. Cut a slit in the potato and press on the ends to open it. Top with black bean chili, salsa, green onions, and cilantro.

Per serving: 376 calories; 11 g protein; 82 g carbohydrate; 0.5 g fat;
450 mg sodium; 0 mg cholesterol

Baked Falafel Sandwich

Makes 20 falafel patties.

Stuff a piece of whole wheat pita bread with these baked falafel patties for a delicious "Middle Eastern Taco."

 1 potato, diced
 1 15-ounce can garbanzo beans, drained
 1 small onion, finely chopped
 ½ cup fresh parsley, chopped fine
 2 garlic cloves, minced
 2 tablespoons tahini (sesame seed butter)
 2 tablespoons soy sauce
 ½ teaspoon turmeric
 ½ teaspoon coriander
 1 teaspoon cumin
 ⅛ teaspoon cayenne
 Pita bread
 Garnishes: lettuce, cucumber, tomato, green onions
 salsa (optional)

Steam the diced potato over boiling water until soft it is about minutes. Place the drained garbanzo beans in a bowl, add the cooked potato, and mash. Add the onion, parsley, garlic, tahini, soy sauce, turmeric, coriander, cumin, and cayenne. Mix well.

Preheat the oven to 350° F. Form the garbanzo mixture into small (walnut-sized) patties and place on a greased baking sheet. Bake for 15 minutes, then turn with a spatula and bake an additional 15 minutes.

Warm the pita bread in foil in the oven, or by steaming it, or heating it briefly in a microwave oven. Stuff two or three falafel patties into the warm pita bread and garish with lettuce, cucumber, tomato, and green onions. Top with salsa if desired.

Per falafel: 214 calories; 8 g protein; 39 g carbohydrate; 2 g fat;
260 mg of sodium; 0 mg carbohydrate

Tip: Fantastic Foods makes an excellent instant falafel mix: just add water and let it stand a few minutes, then form into patties and bake as above.

Pasta with Creamy Pesto

Serves 8

This is pesto that you can enjoy to your heart's content. It's made with silken tofu and contains no added oil.

1 12-ounce package pasta
¼-½ teaspoon salt
1 10.5-ounce package firm silken tofu
2 cups fresh basil leaves
1 garlic clove
½ teaspoon salt

Cook the pasta in boiling water until it is tender, then drain and rinse it. Sprinkle with ¼ teaspoon of salt and toss to mix.

While the pasta is cooking, combine the remaining ingredients in a food processor. Blend until completely smooth, stopping the processor occasionally and scraping down the sides with a rubber spatula.

Add the pesto to the pasta and toss gently to mix. Serve at once.

Per serving: 158 calories; 8 g protein; 28 g carbohydrate; 1 g fat;
204 to 270 mg of sodium; 0 mg cholesterol

Curried Mushrooms and Chickpeas

Serves 8

This spicy Indian dish is delicious with rice or couscous. You can make it hotter or milder by adjusting the amount of cayenne.

½ cup water
2 large onions, chopped
1½ tablespoons cumin seeds
1½ pounds mushrooms, sliced
1 28-ounce can crushed tomatoes
1 15-ounce can garbanzo beans, drained
1 teaspoon turmeric
1 teaspoon coriander
½ teaspoon cayenne
½ teaspoon ginger

Heat the water in a large pot, then add the onions and cook until they are soft. Add the cumin seeds and mushrooms, and continue cooking over medium heat until the mushrooms are light brown.

Add the tomatoes, garbanzo beans, and spices. Cook 30 minutes or longer, until the mushrooms are tender and the flavors are well blended.

Per serving: 116 calories; 5 g protein; 20 g carbohydrate; 1 g fat; 286 mg sodium; 0 mg cholesterol

Ginger Peachy Bread Pudding

Serves 9

1 28-ounce can sliced peaches
1 tablespoon cornstarch
6 cups cubed whole grain bread (about 8 slices)
1¾ cups soy milk or rice milk
⅓ cup packed brown sugar
¾ cup golden raisins
½ teaspoon ginger
½ teaspoon cinnamon
¼ teaspoon nutmeg
¼ teaspoon salt
1 teaspoon vanilla
¼ cup finely chopped crystallized ginger (optional)
2 tablespoons brown sugar

Drain the liquid from the peaches into a large mixing bowl and add the cornstarch. Stir to dissolve any lumps, then add the bread cubes, soy or rice milk, brown sugar, raisins, ginger, cinnamon, nutmeg, salt, and vanilla. Mix well. Stir in the crystallized ginger if desired. Chop the peaches and stir them to the mixture. Spread in a 9 x 9-inch baking dish, then sprinkle the top with brown sugar and let stand 5 minutes while the oven preheats to 350° F. Bake for 35 minutes. Serve warm or cooled.

*Per serving: 252 calories; 3 g protein; 57 g carbohydrate; 1 g fat;
185 mg sodium; 0 mg cholesterol*

Peach Cobbler

Serves 9

Fresh peaches are the essence of summertime, and this is such a delicious way to eat them. If you get a yearning for this cobbler in the middle of winter, use frozen peaches instead.

½ cup sugar
2 tablespoons cornstarch
1 cup water
5 cups sliced peaches, fresh or frozen
½ teaspoon cinnamon
1¼ cups whole wheat pastry flour
2 tablespoons sugar
1½ teaspoons baking powder
¼ teaspoon salt
½ cup soy milk or rice milk

Mix the sugar and cornstarch in a saucepan, then stir in the water and peaches. Bring to a boil and cook over medium-high heat, stirring constantly, until the sauce is clear and thick.

Pour into a 9 x 9-inch baking dish, and sprinkle with the cinnamon. Preheat the oven to 375° F. Mix the flour, 2 tablespoons of sugar, baking powder, and salt in a large bowl, then stir in the soy milk or rice milk to form a batter. Drop by spoonfuls onto the hot peach mixture. Bake until golden brown, about 30 minutes.

Per serving: 178 calories; 3 g protein; 40 g carbohydrate; 0 g fat; 73 mg sodium; 0 mg cholesterol

Chocolate Torte

Serves 12

This torte is pure chocolate decadence. It tastes unbelievably rich, yet is surprisingly low in fat.

In a medium saucepan, stir together the following:

1 cup couscous
1 cup sugar
¼ cup cocoa
¼ teaspoon salt
2½ cups water

Bring to a simmer and cook over medium heat until thickened, about 7 minutes. Spread in the bottom of an ungreased 9-inch springform pan.

In another medium saucepan, combine the following:

½ cup sugar
5 tablespoons cornstarch
3 tablespoons cocoa
2 cups soy milk or rice milk

Whisk smooth, then cook over medium heat, stirring constantly until very thick (like thick pudding). Spread evenly over the top of the couscous mixture.

Refrigerate until set, at least 2 hours, before serving.

Per serving (¹⁄₁₂ th of pie): 161 calories; 3 g protein;
36 g carbohydrate; 1 g fat; 106 mg sodium; 0 mg cholesterol

Gingerbread

Makes 9 2-inch pieces

1⅔ cups unbleached or whole wheat pastry flour
1 teaspoons baking soda
½ teaspoon salt
1½ teaspoons cinnamon
1½ teaspoons ginger
1 10.5-ounce package firm silken tofu
½ cup sugar
¼ cup molasses
½ cup raisins

Preheat oven to 375⁰ F. Mix the flour, baking soda, salt, cinnamon, and ginger in a large bowl.

Place the tofu, sugar, and molasses into a food processor and blend until completely smooth. Add to the flour mixture and stir until just blended. Mix in the raisins. Spread in an oil-sprayed 8-inch square baking dish, and bake in the preheated oven for 25 minutes. Use a spatula to loosen the gingerbread from the pan, then turn it out onto a rack to cool.

Per muffin: 198 calories; 6 g protein; 41 g carbohydrate; 1 g fat; 224 mg sodium; 0 mg cholesterol

Banana Freeze

Serves 2

Frozen bananas make a thick and creamy dessert with no added fat. To freeze the bananas, peel and break them into pieces. Place them loosely in a covered container to freeze.

½ cup soy milk or rice milk
4-6 pitted dates
2 cups frozen banana chunks
1 teaspoon vanilla

Place the soy milk and dates into a blender and blend until the dates are in very small pieces. Add the bananas and vanilla.

Blend on high speed until thick and smooth, stopping the blender to stir any unblended fruit to the center.

Per serving: 143 calories; 3 g protein; 30 g carbohydrate; 1 g fat; 46 mg of sodium; 0 mg cholesterol

Index